THE

INCREDIBLE

SHRINKING

CRITIC

ALSO BY JAMI BERNARD

Breast Cancer: There & Back

*The X List: The National Society of Film Critics'
Guide to Movies That Turn Us On*
(editor)

*Chick Flicks: The Movie Lover's Guide
to the Movies Women Love*

Quentin Tarantino: The Man and His Movies

Total Exposure

*First Films: Illustrious, Obscure and
Embarrassing Movie Debuts*

75 Pounds and Counting:

AVERY

a member of

Penguin Group (USA) Inc.

New York

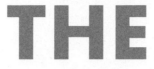

THE
INCREDIBLE
SHRINKING
CRITIC

My Excellent Adventure in Weight Loss

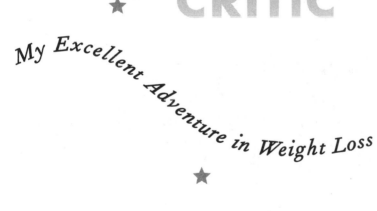

JAMI
BERNARD

AVERY

Published by the Penguin Group
Penguin Group (USA) Inc., 375 Hudson Street, New York, New York 10014, USA •
Penguin Group (Canada), 90 Eglinton Avenue East, Suite 700, Toronto, Ontario M4P 2Y3, Canada
(a division of Pearson Penguin Canada Inc.) • Penguin Books Ltd, 80 Strand, London WC2R 0RL,
England • Penguin Ireland, 25 St Stephen's Green, Dublin 2, Ireland (a division of Penguin Books Ltd) •
Penguin Group (Australia), 250 Camberwell Road, Camberwell, Victoria 3124, Australia (a division of
Pearson Australia Group Pty Ltd) • Penguin Books India Pvt Ltd, 11 Community Centre, Panchsheel
Park, New Delhi–110 017, India • Penguin Group (NZ), Cnr Airborne and Rosedale Roads, Albany,
Auckland 1310, New Zealand (a division of Pearson New Zealand Ltd) • Penguin Books
(South Africa) (Pty) Ltd, 24 Sturdee Avenue, Rosebank, Johannesburg 2196, South Africa

Penguin Books Ltd, Registered Offices: 80 Strand, London WC2R 0RL, England

Most Avery books are available at special quantity discounts for bulk purchase for sales promotions, premiums, fund-raising, and educational needs. Special books or book excerpts also can be created to fit specific needs. For details, write Penguin Group (USA) Inc. Special Markets, 375 Hudson Street, New York, NY 10014.

Library of Congress Cataloging-in-Publication Data
Bernard, Jami.
The incredible shrinking critic : 75 pounds and counting : my excellent
adventure in weight loss / by Jami Bernard
p.   cm.
Includes index.
ISBN 1-58333-262-6
1. Bernard, Jami—Health.   2. Overweight women—United States—Biography.
3. Weight loss—Case studies.   I. Title.
RC628.B399   2006   2006042967
362.196'3980092—dc22
[B]

Printed in the United States of America
1   3   5   7   9   10   8   6   4   2

BOOK DESIGN BY MEIGHAN CAVANAUGH

While the author has made every effort to provide accurate telephone numbers and Internet addresses at the time of publication, neither the publisher nor the author assumes any responsibility for errors, or for changes that occur after publication. Further, the publisher does not have any control over and does not assume any responsibility for author or third-party websites or their content.

This is not a book of professional advice, but one woman's story about her personal battle to lose weight. The ideas, procedures, and suggestions contained in this book that worked for the author may not be suitable for you. All matters regarding your health require medical supervision, and before embarking on any diet program, you should consult with your personal physician. Neither the author nor the publisher shall be liable or responsible for any loss or damage allegedly arising from any information or suggestion in this book.

The recipes contained in this book are to be followed exactly as written. The publisher is not responsible for your specific health or allergy needs that may require medical supervision. The publisher is not responsible for any adverse reactions to the recipes contained in this book.

To Terry and Diane . . .

for taking me in

and showering me

with love

CONTENTS

Part Two

★

The Knack, and How to Get It

PREFACE
PIZZA FOR LIFE

The fellow who owned the pizza place was a bit of a celebrity in my neighborhood. He was a fixture, a family man, so I won't antagonize his brick-oven heirs by naming him.

He didn't do anything wrong, technically speaking, but he'd sigh and stare exaggerated sighs, glassy-eyed stares— whenever I stopped by his parlor for a slice.

Which was often.

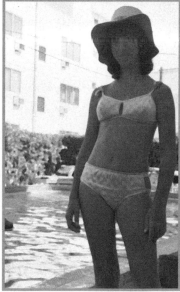

One afternoon when I was about twelve and beginning to bud in all the right places, the pizza man served up a slice and wouldn't take my money. "Your body, it's just ... *all there*," he sighed. It was tight, it was right. He shook his head as if to say, *Who can grasp such ineffable wonders?* Then he offered me a deal.

At twelve, budding just enough to merit free pizza.

xiii

"If I could have just one night with you, I'd give you free pizza for life."

I giggled and blushed. But my mind was racing; *I wanted the pizza*. One roll in the dough didn't seem too much to ask.

Sex for pizza, the bottomless pie! Let's see, that's 15 cents a slice, a few times a week . . . for life! He was thinking sex, I was thinking food.

I responded to the pizza man the way I respond (even today) to many offers over which I'm conflicted—I stiffened in embarrassed confusion like a Madame Tussaud exhibit. By the time I came up with a clever rejoinder, one designed to send the man away while subtly keeping my options open, the moment had passed, the pizza man had moved on down the counter.

He didn't forget me, though. He renewed his sex-for-pizza offer every time I came in, until I sheepishly found another pizza place, half as good and half a mile away, simply to avoid the discomfort of a sexually charged situation that was interfering with my enjoyment of those hot, stretchy strands of melted cheese.

My body might have been saying, *Hey, sailor!*, but at twelve, I was still a child. I liked biking and paddleball. I'd stumbled upon the joys of Dirty Barbie at age nine (Ken saves Barbie from drowning at the beach but her zebra-striped maillot falls off!), but actual sex was still far off the radar. It would be another year before my first date—ice skating in Central Park followed by an awkward peck with teeth clenched. And it would be what seemed like a lifetime before I lost my virginity to a boy who was so nervous he had to run a comb through his hair first.

But think of the pizza I could have had! Maybe he'd have thrown in some slices of Sicilian!

Food and sex. Food and men. Food, sex, men. What a mess. I never wanted it to be this way, but that's how life unfolded—all appetites and desires led somehow to romantic disappointment, then to rage; last stop, Twinkies. In my mid-thirties, when I no longer danced the calories off at after-hours clubs, the slow creep of pudge became a mud slide. Weight gain was a result of many interlocking factors—cluelessness, careless-ness, sybaritic indulgence—but also, I think, a subconscious effort to in-sulate myself with a literal wall of fat. Looking less desirable would make my bosses take me seriously, stop men from whispering sick things to me on the street, keep female friends from being competitive and jealous.

It didn't work! I got fat all right, but now my bosses ignored me, rivals turned contemptuous, and the physical padding didn't protect me from romantic misadventure after all. It just made me buy hideous clothes.

I decided to take a hard look at myself. No wonder those diets I'd tried from time to time hadn't worked, or at least hadn't worked for long; on some level I *wanted* to be fat. What I needed was a new security blanket, one not pegged to food. Or perhaps I was ready to chuck the security blankets and stop living my life in free-floating fear.

Self-knowledge is a rocky road that doesn't guarantee weight loss. At the same time, I knew I was through with diets. They all suck, on a slid-ing scale of suckage. When I was ready to lose weight I did it the old-fashioned way—through eating responsibly, changing habits, becoming more active. This could only come about by rethinking how I ate and thought about food, in addition to rethinking myself from the ground up; losing the weight depended on a balance of all these components, not just one alone. I chronicled the process publicly in a weekly column in the New York *Daily News*, where I worked thirteen years as a movie critic, about as sedentary a job as there is. (Sit for two hours in the dark, sit for two hours at the computer. Back to the theater, back to the computer. Then lunch.)

There was no rush. I didn't have to wriggle into a particular pair of jeans on a chosen weekend. But I had a specific goal, an umbrella goal that encompassed dozens of smaller ones. It was a goal I'd fiddled with idly, mostly subconsciously, until the day I stepped on the scale and was aston-ished to see: *I weighed 230 pounds.*

I decided to lose 100 pounds. This is the story of how I lost 75 of them.

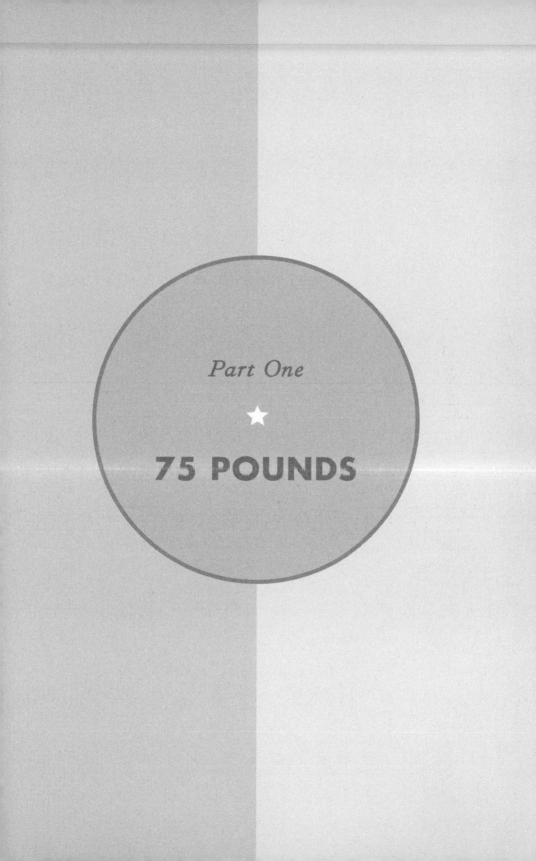

Part One

★

75 POUNDS

HOPPING THE KETTLE

I didn't see it coming. Really, I didn't. I awoke like Kafka's Gregor Samsa to find myself transformed, not into a gigantic bug, but into . . . *a big ol' fat person*. The former disco baby who had danced all night at Studio 54 and had men taking numbers was gone, encased—perhaps like a candy's creamy center—within the body of a woman who weighed . . . considerably more.

I awoke to find I weighed 230 pounds. Or I should say, I finally opened my eyes to it, which is very different, because there's knowing and there's *knowing*. The extra weight didn't arrive overnight, but I was the proverbial frog in the slowly heating pot that acclimates to the temperature and thus is complicit in its own death.

Actually—and here's good news for the frog—Victor Hutchison at the University of Oklahoma's zoology department proved that an amphibian's "critical thermal maxima" will goad it into making increasingly frantic attempts to get the hell out. I shudder to think how Dr. Hutchison went about this experiment. But I know I reached my own critical thermal

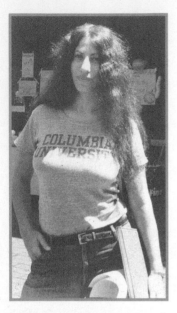

I still see myself as I was in college, even though this particular picture was taken on a "fat" day, wearing the Fat Pants of yesteryear. *(Photo by Matthew Nemerson)*

maxima at 230 pounds, and although I'd attempted to hop the kettle many times—a financial boon for gyms, spas, and weight-loss programs across Manhattan—this time I made it over the rim.

I lost the weight. No foods were demonized, no fads embraced, no frogs boiled.

I charted my initial weight loss in the *Daily News,* where the editor in chief du jour came up with the column's title: "Our Incredible Shrinking Critic!" I would have curled up under a desk with shame, but when you're fat it's difficult to curl at all, and in tabloid journalism you never say no, even when your editors are determined to make you look like an idiot, so I waddled forth into the public spotlight week after week under that feverish banner.

It was a daring or foolhardy move, depending on your perspective. To make up for the denial in which I'd basked for so long, my body was out there on display for a million readers. If I failed, which is what usually happens when people publicly announce they're going to quit smoking or lose weight or stop skimming profits from their company, it would be a very public splat.

There's nothing like the prospect of major humiliation to organize a person. I had no intention of failing. And I had no idea what was coming.

It was exhilarating. It was a nightmare. The first time the column ran, I was reluctant to go outdoors. When I did, I was afraid to be seen shopping, not even for lettuce. As the column progressed, I was frequently recognized on the street, in stores, on the subway. At the beginning it was weird, then kind of a kick. I learned to tamp down my inclination when stared at to respond with the New Yorker's ever-ready *Whatchoo lookin' at?*

Readers responded to the column because it was written on the tightrope walk of real time. Unlike media splashes that show quick, stupendous weight loss but never follow up to see how those miracle slimmers are doing a few months later, my column doggedly acknowledged the jagged, uncertain graph that represents the true face of weight loss. Legions of unsung weight losers wrote in, recognizing their own struggles in my infinitesimal victories over fractions of pounds. A critic at a rival paper sent me a juicy tribute: a box of Harry & David's pears.

There were also people who thought the column unseemly, too personal. Even in the age of reality TV, this was too . . . *real*. Naked, even. One of my editors, a fat chick herself who nevertheless insisted on wearing midriff blouses to the office, glared daggers at me whenever we passed. Society's simmering fear and hatred of fat often spills over into revulsion of individuals who carry it on their hips. While some readers wanted to date me (and were quite insistent), others were furious. They didn't know me, yet they hated me. Was it because I was fat? Because I was getting thinner? Both? Perhaps they were peeved that I dared go about my life either way, fat or thin, insufficiently apologetic about taking up space in their world. There are those who take comfort in assuming that fat people think only of their fat, the way sighted people think the blind ruminate unceasingly on their blindness. My weight bothered some strangers more than it bothered me, though I doubt they had my health and well-being in mind.

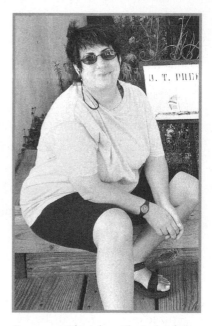

Greenport: This is how I looked right before reaching critical thermal maxima. *(Photo by Donna Dickman)*

One reader insisted I was too fat for

him to bear to read my column, yet he followed it breathlessly, scrutiniz-ing it for slipups, reaffirming his boycott via regular e-mails, his anger growing in inverse proportion to my body mass index. He seemed vio-lated by my weight loss, as if he had a stake in it. It's not unusual for com-plete strangers to feel irrational fury over other people's bodies; dime-store psychology has it that they're secretly terrified it could happen to them.

And, of course, it can.

★

I carried it well, as they say. Most people had no idea I was anywhere near the 200 mark. Until those final 10 or 20 pounds, my face remained rela-tively slender, my body proportional. In TV appearances, as long as they shot me head-on, I could pass.

My flesh was tight, muscles compact. My first personal trainer, Nor-man, told me I had the body of a weight lifter—not the compliment I was hoping for (what, no ballerina neck?), yet something to take pride in nev-ertheless. I'm no athlete, but I wasn't *soft*-fat, I was hard-fat. Like those thin people who anxiously reassure themselves that at least they're not *fat*, I too congratulated myself that at least I wasn't *that* fat, not *sloppy* fat. My ass not as wide as that one there, my chin not doubled like this one here. Being fat doesn't necessarily qualify you for Humanitarian of the Year; you still gauge yourself against everyone else and find murky re-serves of smugness. We all need a safe divide between *them* and *us,* and the illusion that we're somehow superior for it.

I carried it well. Still, no one mistook me for merely "overweight," as I delicately described myself. My mother, with typical dramatic embel-lishment, confided to my sister that she thought I was 300 pounds.

I was asked after the fact whether I'd ever considered surgery. Cer-tainly not; I truly wasn't *that* fat. My health wasn't in imminent danger.

My cholesterol, blood pressure, ratio of "good" fat to bad, all aspects of my bloodwork are spectacular—a crazy, welcome gift of genetics. (Don't worry, genetics got me in other areas.) Plus, surgery is too extreme if you haven't exhausted safer routes, like—*hello!*—eating right, exercising, and, in my case, making an honest appraisal of how and why I'd gotten so fat after a rail-thin childhood and wasp-waisted early adulthood.

My youth had been active and social, with boyfriends and fun. (Maybe too much fun.) I still carried myself with the sense memory of my healthy-weight twenties. Why and where had I sucked up all that fat? As my doorman once said in alarm after seeing a photo of the old me running a race in Central Park, *"What did you do to yourself?"* (No holiday tip for him.)

When I finally allowed my mind to drift to the possibility of hunkering down and losing weight, I realized that despite previous efforts to that end, whose souvenirs included folders of officially stamped attendance cards from Weight Watchers and nutrition books fluttering with Post-its where I'd marked important passages, and despite years of intermittent spa-cuisine classes and abs crunches, I'd never made a concerted, serious effort to lose weight. I hadn't devoted nearly the time, resources, or enthusiasm to losing weight that I had to finding the perfect cat toy. (Tsuko is very particular.)

There was no time for the gym—perish the thought—but there was always time in the margins to write a book, putter around, take up a new hobby. Like everyone I know, I'd been laboring under the impression that there was no fat in the schedule for exercise or the myriad things you need to concentrate on to rev up a healthy lifestyle. The problem was that I hadn't been willing to make my body a priority; apparently, I hadn't wanted to, and the reasons were buried in layers of internal muck.

If the first great shock was seeing 230 on the scale—and that was shock enough—the second was that I'd been kidding myself. And if I was kidding myself about my weight and priorities, what else was I hiding from myself? I wanted to know. I wanted to know *everything* about myself, including what other people saw when they looked at me.

When you open the door to the self, it's like that moment in *The Amityville Horror* when the house screams hoarsely, *Get out!* Some of what I learned made me want to jump back in the pot with the frog. My friend JoAnne admitted that sometimes I can be a pill. My sister said there were times I'd acted like "a monster," and that Mom and Dad changed the locks after I went off to college.

Monster? Er . . . how did my parents get that impression? But now that I think of it, the immigrant news vendor on my corner once screamed at me, "Fuck you, Miss!" He must have had a reason.

It turns out that not all my behavior has been stellar. Sure, I'm good-hearted, funny, empathetic, and genuine. Then there's that little matter of when I'm selfish, hostile, petty, and melancholy. Knowing your real self can be quite a letdown. And once you're on to yourself, there's an implicit responsibility to change for the better; what a drag *that* is. I should stop being selfish? What's in it for *me?*

It was unpleasant at times. But I frankly couldn't have lost the weight without all that soul searching or whatever you want to call it: navel-gazing, self-actualization, a fantastic voyage up your own butt—yes, to the heart of darkness! The dream of self-improvement is integral to the American spirit, which explains all those boozy, bleary New Year's resolutions like "Be a better person."

Self-knowledge is a bitch. No wonder the urge to seek it usually wears off by mimosa time at the New Year's Day brunch.

Still, the journey was worth it. Weight loss is commonly measured in numbers, but losing 75 pounds turned out to be secondary to self-knowledge, which can't be quantified. To live healthfully isn't just about eating right and getting enough sleep, it's also about being in harmony with yourself—and I don't mean that in a mystical sense. All the diets in the world couldn't have pried the fat from my hips until I understood how and why I'd laid it on in the first place. My fat might have been screaming, *Feed me!* But it was also screaming, *You need me!*

Sharing this inner journey as it occurred wasn't always easy, but such a challenge can be fun, even addictive, like a reality show where they perform a makeover on your psyche. Lose the metaphorical chintz! As I chipped away at the mental blocks, I also learned to eat better and live better. The weight dropped off in teeny, tiny increments.

Many of my readers were inspired to lose weight along with me. They helped me by offering e-mail encouragement, and I reciprocated with advice and information from experts in the field. In this book, I'll also share all that with you, even Roger Ebert's recipe for rice-cooker oatmeal. He swears by it—oatmeal for breakfast and a pedometer on the belt. But enough about Roger.

During a routine checkup, my oncologist warned me in unusually frank terms—he used the five-letter "o" word, which shall not pass my lips—that by continuing to gain weight, I was courting a recurrence of the breast cancer I'd battled successfully in 1996.

Much of my weight gain came from a misguided attempt to soothe myself with food in the wake of surgery, chemo, and radiation; you can't blame a cancer survivor for clinging to the Ben & Jerry's lifeboat. I well knew that estrogen-rich abdominal fat has been linked in some studies to increased risk of breast cancer, but I'd compartmentalized the problem as something to take care of one day when I was "ready," as if awaiting a sudden sprinkling of low-cal pixie dust, after which everything would be made right.

Every extra pound tells a story. It's a story of anger, frustration, old wounds, and carelessness. It's a story of misjudged portions, too-hasty celebrations, bad planning, misplaced optimism. It's a story of denial.

Every pound also cost a small fortune. I was paying for ever-expansive clothing, gym memberships and diet food, weight-management seminars and spa vacations, talk therapy, behavior therapy, personal trainers. I'd lose some weight, buy clothing in anticipation of a smaller size, then gain back the weight (and more) while the new wardrobe hung in the closet with the tags still on.

I'll bet each extra pound ultimately cost me $1,000.

I'd give anything to lose weight, I'd think. Right. Anything except inconvenience myself.

It's not like I'm lazy! I'd ask myself in exasperation, Just what is the *problem* here? I'm a high achiever, I'm motivated. Even driven. I love weight training, biking, swimming. After cancer, I took up skiing and horseback riding just for fun. I'm a hard worker. I go the extra mile. (I just don't go the extra mile in sweatpants.)

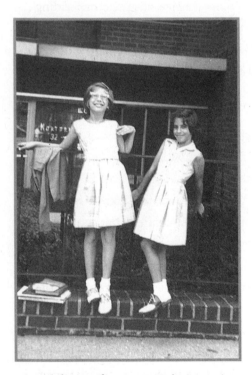

Diane (left) mugs for camera. We're in our sister dresses. (*Photo by Sam Bernard*)

Was there something intrinsically wrong with me? Could I blame my ancestors, who looked alarmingly sturdy in photos taken at Brighton Beach back in the day? My older sister and I had been skinny kids, but even though I'm relatively athletic, while my sister is proud of having conserved her energy like a milk-fed veal calf, we wound up only a few pounds apart by our early forties. It's as if we'd been identically programmed.

I didn't hate myself. But I hated being fat. It's an important distinction: Hate the sin, not the sinner.

Shopping for clothes was depressing; don't bring any sharp objects with you to department-store fitting rooms. Typical styles for the overweight favor cheery constellations of rhinestones, huge flowers, or loud prints that scream, *Hello! I come from the Planet Fat and I mean you no harm!*

Humiliation was everywhere. At the relatively slender weight of 170 I was dating a man who would smugly announce after dinner, "I see you're a member of the Clean Plate Club again!" At least that's what I *think* he said. The sound waves had trouble making it around his gigantic beer gut.

At a local stable, the only horse they'd let me ride was Boulder, the brute reserved for Paul Bunyan's descendants. The receptionist squinted disbelievingly at my application, then yelled—in front of a gaggle of beanpole ladies who were adjusting their form-fitting, tailored riding pants—*"How much did you say you weigh, dear?"*

When you're the fattest person on a horse or taking a gym class or in a pool, it would be great if everyone looked on with encouragement and admiration: "Bless my soul, Muffy, that girl may be fat, but she's *doing something about it! I applaud her!*"

That's not how it went down. Muffy would regard me with alarm, as if my cellulite were spoiling her view. I took up space, *her* space. I didn't belong in the public arena.

I've been fat and I've been thin. So I know firsthand that there's a big, fat difference in how people respond to you depending on your size. When you're thin, you get more respect whether you deserve it or not. When you're fat, people look right through you as if you don't exist—if you're lucky. Otherwise, they act as if you've personally offended them. They assume you're fat because you're stupid, lazy, and morally bankrupt, as if you made a choice one day: *You know, I think I'll get really fat so I'll suffer health problems, have trouble finding a job, be the butt of jokes and cruelty, court diabetes, endure society's wrath, and die young. That's the life for me!*

A reader wrote in to ask, How does an otherwise intelligent person get so fat?

Putting aside for the moment that this reader should be boiled in a pot *with a lid,* he poses a question that's on a lot of minds. America is getting tubbier by the minute—except in a few documented places like New Hampshire (do they shiver off the pounds?). About 65 percent of the country is overweight or worse. (You know, that other "o" word.)

So many fat folk. Yet the perception still clings that it's a class issue— that fat means unsophisticated, a predilection for nonbreathable synthetic fabrics. Only the poor and uneducated Mayors McCheese of the nation would "let themselves go," their jowly faces lighting up at Big Gulps and Double-Doubles, the type who offend the very eyeballs of proper citizens.

What short memories. Fat weaves in and out of fashion, and once upon a time, it was a sign of status, visible proof of a stocked larder. Only the rich (think of the ruddy-faced royalty of yore sporting the festering wounds of gout) could afford to parade about with flesh on their bones. Not until recent times has fat come to represent the stigma of poverty. Food became cheap and plentiful (at least in America, the capital of eating disorders), while medical advances prolonged life so that gauntness no longer automatically connoted plague or a wasting disease. The rich changed tactics and began to set themselves apart from the masses with a new display of wealth—thinness—as if to say, I don't need to get my money's worth at an all-you-can-eat buffet. I can afford to be thin.

Personally, I believe so many rich people are thin because they can afford lobster. Lobster has so few calories—90 of them per 3½ ounces, as opposed to 280 calories for the same amount of steak—it's practically like eating iceberg lettuce all day.

At no time soon will our culture lose the idea that fat is for the less deserving, even though it's an equal-opportunity debaser, attaching to random inner thighs without first checking wallets or SAT scores. Rich or poor, if you're using food to stanch emotional wounds, the only thing that can make you feel better on the spot—and this is a scientific fact—is cheese fries.

★

My discomfort had been growing, the pot simmering. Months before I hit 230, I began to entertain the notion that it was possible, theoretically, to lose 100 pounds. Not 83 pounds, not 105 pounds, but 100, a nice round figure, the roundest of figures, like my own. The number stuck in my mind and my craw. I made it personally meaningful, imbuing it with majesty, because deep down I was searching for something vivid to galvanize me. *One hundred pounds*—such an important number, profound, meaty, balanced—perfect in its way, with those mystical zeroes.

The number was specific, yet the idea was an abstraction. I'm not sure I thought it applied to me at all, just that losing 100 pounds would be a dramatic and exciting thing for *someone* to do.

Without realizing it, I was getting ready, moving like a bullet into the chamber.

When reason fails, there's shock. I was jolted from that miasma of

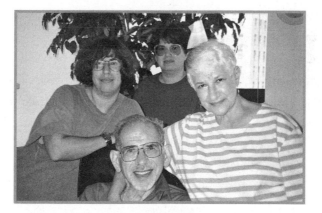

From top left clockwise: Me, Diane, Mom, Dad. At least Mom could still wear horizontal stripes. Here I look 20 pounds heavier than I was, thanks to bad clothing, haircut, posture.

what addiction literature calls "pre-contemplation" by an irreconcilable disconnect between how I perceived myself and what I weighed. I'd look in the mirror and see . . . I don't know what I saw. Maybe nothing, a vampire without reflection. I had no clear idea what I looked like, what I weighed, what size I was. It wasn't displeasure or self-hate or any recognizable emotion, just an absence. I was blinded by denial as the disparity grew between how I viewed myself—the seductive disco baby who never waited in line at Studio 54 (the press pass helped) and was deserving of free pizza, the bottomless pie—and what the mirror said (if only I could register it). When I looked in the mirror, it was as if I focused a centimeter past the glass to the silver backing beyond.

When the great schism occurred—the I Can't Take It Any More moment, set off by the repellent number 230 on the digital scale—my phoenix rose from the ashes.

My phoenix might have plopped right back into bed, ashes and all, if I hadn't been marinating sufficiently all along in the preparation stage, mentally rehearsing for weight loss. By the time my phoenix took flight, I already knew what I needed to do, and, equally important, I had a general idea of how to go about it. You can itch for action all you want, but without a game plan you'll probably retreat in frustration or settle for a fad diet that has you eating cabbage on alternate Wednesdays (but only if you're a Libra).

You can certainly lose some weight on *any* diet, but this book isn't about fitting into a micromini by Saturday or worrying that your Brazilian bikini wax doesn't show to best advantage. If you're whining over your final five pounds, suck in your gut and go on your way. Leave the rest of us to serious weight loss, the kind that requires a reasonable, long-term strategy and at least a vague comprehension that the ultimate goal is change, not the superficial goal of an arbitrary number. This book is about big-time weight loss—losing it for good—where each pound must be untangled from a fusion of benign neglect and self-destructive habit.

Ultimate self-improvement is about changing yourself, not just losing weight.

Now a word about "willpower." Remove it from your vocabulary. Losing serious weight has nothing whatsoever to do with that all-purpose buzzword that implies you're fat because you're a degenerate good-for-nothing. People hurl that word like a gauntlet—*Sir, you lack willpower! Pistols at dawn!*

It doesn't mean you're absolved of complicity in your weight gain. You opened your mouth, you chewed, you swallowed. But medical research and the consensus of experts refutes the "willpower" theory: *Lasting weight loss is about strategy, not willpower.*

Fat people aren't weak-willed—they're willing to starve themselves! But the garden-variety dieter doesn't know the difference between smart planning and running at a brick wall. You can be fiercely determined to steal away Maria Sharapova's endorsement deals, but that doesn't mean you can make a New Year's resolution to compete at Wimbledon the next day. Your indomitable will is no substitute for years of training and practice.

More important, Wimbledon is closed New Year's Day.

Straining to summon diet willpower is like going to Wimbledon the moment you feel the urge to bat a tennis ball around: all ambition, no fundamentals. Any time you feel that internal struggle where willpower dukes it out with a lovely ramekin of molten chocolate cake, it's almost certainly because of a failure to plan ahead for contingencies.

While losing weight, I bumped up against contingencies galore: special occasions, changes in plans, unforeseen circumstances. I remember—oh, how I remember!—a tray of frosted cupcakes at a movie premiere. My friend Eddie Berganza was my date for the evening. My focus kept drifting to the gently peaked cupcakes, their shellacked frosting glistening with come-hither beads of condensation. Eddie cupped his hands around his mouth like a megaphone: *"Step away from the cupcakes!"*

I didn't have a cupcake that night. I went home and instead opened a labor-intensive pomegranate, savoring its pearly, red-stained delights. But I continued to obsess over that party tray in the coming week—a bruised memory, as if that cupcake had ditched me at the altar, leaving me love-starved. It had been a case of willpower winning out over craving; the "willpower" contingent would call that a victory. But the incident was more of a slip. I had forgotten to stick to basics: Don't *ever* go to a party hungry. Don't *ever* loiter near the finger food. When you're raging out of control for whatever reason—hormones, Mars in retrograde, electroshock gone wrong—don't go to the party at all. There's no one rule that suits every occasion, but there's a battery of strategic options, and I'd embarked on that evening totally unarmed, unprepared, defenseless.

The "willpower" people imagine all of weight loss as an epic Battle of the Cupcakes. But with rational weight loss, the kind where you're eating sensibly and living right, willpower sleeps in its basket by the fire, snoring gently.

The typical diet mentality encourages such Battles of the Cupcakes. I know that mentality well, since like just about every female (and half the males) in America I've been on diets before, a card-carrying member of the yo-yo dieters' club. I know the secrets of the yo-yo sisterhood. Some diet plans are better than others, naturally. But they're not designed to address the thornier problems of weight loss. They wouldn't want to, because the more general the program the larger the pool of prospective customers, and to protect themselves from legal issues they hardly want to scoop up those with serious psychological or medical issues. Weight Watchers claims they'll take only people who need to lose 10 pounds or more, so as to discourage anorexics and the like, but I know many women who've rejoined obsessively for those last few sticky pounds.

Commercial diets cannot possibly accommodate every individual's needs, and it's not in their long-term interests to do so—who, then, would buy their products? They needn't worry, because they all have spectacularly high (though largely unreported) recidivism rates.

It's not that commercial diets are necessarily unhealthy (although some are). It's that they are shortsighted, perhaps necessarily so. Plans that sell you prepackaged foods are convenient, but Jenny Craig can't very well hover over you in your kitchen when you finally attempt to feed yourself on your own. Meeting-based plans like Weight Watchers dispense thoughtful behavioral tips that are useless if you're not ready to change or don't know how to get ready to be ready. Rule-based diets like Atkins, the ones that urge you to suck the marrow after polishing off a giant T-bone but to run for your life if you see (*eek!*) a carrot, are impossible to stick to, let alone that their "scientific" rationales don't hold up in the big picture of health. Rule-based plans can be soothing at first, giving disordered eating a sense of order, but most people can't and won't follow tricky subsets of rules for life.

Most of these plans attach a surcharge, whether they mean to or not—they dish up a ruinous diet mentality that hurts your chances of long-term success: *It's all or nothing, baby!*

So first it's all. Then it's nothing.

★ Yo-yo dieting

Bad news for fans of passing the buck: Despite the prevailing wisdom, yo-yo dieting does *not*, after all, ruin your metabolism like an overstretched rubber band.

The idea gained currency after a 1986 study on rats whose weights yo-yo'd after an enforced deprivation diet. Newer studies have failed to confirm those findings; however, studies indicate that yo-yo dieting damages the immune system, depleting it of cells that fight off viruses and cancer.

I took that swan dive into the diet du jour on many occasions. This time was different. The notion of losing 100 pounds gnawed at me for months; I slept on it, chewed on it, the idea burrowing into my mind and heart, an earthworm aerating my subconscious. There's no one particular day on which I embraced losing weight, only a gradual understanding that it was possible and would entail changing everything.

So the idea to lose weight, the commitment to it, the readiness, came way before the scale hit a number that gave me such pain I couldn't reconcile it with the vision of my younger self breezing past the ropes at Studio 54.

How, then, did I take action, if not by joining the devotees of the Fatkins plan as they marched to their future coronaries?

I started my weight loss with a big bowl of pasta and a glass of wine.

2

THE FIRST 10:
THE MIRROR CRACK'D

There's a Sufi tale I love. Like all Sufi tales, it's a shaggy-dog story that takes forever to tell, so I'll just sum up: Man wants wisdom, asks bum where to find the Sufi master on the mount. Bum says, "Thataway." Man travels—miles, years, whatever. Runs into bum again; "Thataway." Mountains, deserts, valleys. Man finally climbs mount, finds Sufi master—and he turns out to be the bum! The rags and tatters have turned to robes of glistening gold! "Hey, bum, why didn't you tell me it was you all along?" asks the man, pissed off. And the wise old Sufi explains, "You were not ready to recognize me."

If anyone had asked me if I wanted to lose weight, I'd have said yes. But oh, I had to travel hills and dales and pass many bums until I was ready to do so.

Isaac Newton was probably thinking of me when he stated his first law of motion, the one about how an object at rest tends to stay that way. What he meant was that a person who eats cake for breakfast will continue to do so until bakeries go out of business. We don't seek change until our world is rocked. Close encounters of the mortal kind—a heart attack or other health crisis—are often an effective wake-up call, at least for those who wake up. After I had breast cancer, I went vegan for six months. But the memory and immediacy of those chemo injections dissipated over time, and soon I was back to using food recklessly, which for me was as foolish as operating heavy machinery on NyQuil.

You can lose some weight even when you're not totally committed to it. But for major weight loss and long-term results, you need the click. Gotta have the click.

Most people who successfully lose weight report a click, a turning point. One minute, losing weight seems impossible, unthinkable. You'd rather go down fighting with a piping hot, lightly salted, tender-crisp clutch of fries in your defiant fist.

The next minute, you're the Zen master of weight loss. O frabjous day! Callooh! Callay!

The click comes and goes, seemingly miraculous and elusive. When it hits, it precipitates ecstatic plunges into diets and calorie counting, with loved ones cheering you on as if you're running the last lap of the Olympic flame relay. Yet the enthusiasm can fade in the time it takes to lick the white off an Oreo. You're in mid-lick and the moment has passed, darkness falls. You can hardly recall your past life as someone who ate—and enjoyed—bran flakes. There is only now, and a sleeve of Oreos.

This time around, my click arrived in the form of a number—230. It was . . . unacceptable. Grotesque. I don't know why 229 had been any better, but that's an epiphany for ya.

In a huge, ongoing study of successful weight losers, 75 percent experienced a triggering event. The epiphany usually arrives in a moment of intense discomfort. It can be the physical pain of a heart attack or the mental dissonance between how you see yourself and how you look in that unspeakable photo from your cousin's wedding, where you were planted like a gag prop among bridesmaids in single-digit-sized dresses with spaghetti straps.

You wouldn't want to go out of your way to bring on a heart attack just so you can be shocked back into health, and anyway, the shock as it unfolds usually feels random and beyond control. But you can synthetically recreate that moment of clarity in your very own petri dish of behavior. (Here we're talking advanced coursework; see Part 2, Chapter 1 for details.)

Generally speaking, most people won't get to the click until they're shocked into it. I have a close friend whose head is always in the clouds. To get through to him, you practically have to clap cymbals over his head, after which he'll blink and say, "Well, *that* got my attention!"

The number 230 got my attention. I'd had epiphanies before, but this one was different. It felt less . . . circumstantial.

There's no substitution for that feeling of sudden, intense epiphany. But the common wisdom that it's a switch—either on or off—is a misconception. Weight loss is a process, a plodding one at that. The epiphany isn't what makes you ready to lose weight, it's the other way around: When you're in a state of readiness, you see the light.

Readiness comes by degrees. It might feel like a sudden revelation, but it's been building inside you, and there's nothing mysterious about it: The readiness to change destructive habits has been quantified through parallel research on cigarette and alcohol addictions. It's called "stages of change," and it's routinely applied to such problem behaviors as unhealthy eating. It's a five-step process, not unlike Elisabeth Kübler-Ross's five stages of grief. Both models begin with denial (here called "precontemplation").

- Stage 1: Pre-contemplation. Might think about the problem, might not.

- Stage 2: Contemplation. I'm thinking, I'm thinking.
- Stage 3: Preparation: What time is that Overeaters Anonymous meeting again?
- Stage 4: Action: "Waiter, sauce on the side."
- Stage 5: Maintenance: I think I'll skip that cupcake party tonight, honey.

The part we think of as readiness to lose weight is the fourth step, action. And the important thing to know is that the magical click people feel when they're ready is simply evidence of movement along this contin-

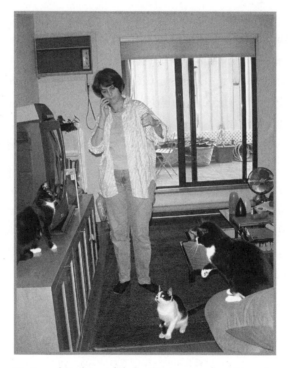

Marie multitasking while bunking at my place. Here she telecommutes while dangling a wand toy for Tsuko (left), Buzz, and Sylvia. *(Photo by Jamie Bernard)*

uum of attitude changes. When you move from Stage 3, preparation, to Stage 4, action, *that's* when you feel the click.

So I clicked. And I began losing weight that very first night with a big bowl of pasta and a glass of wine.

It wasn't one of those all-you-can-eat binges the night before embarking on a deprivation diet. That heaping bowl of pasta with vegetables and seafood was the start of my master plan to lose 100 pounds, slowly and naturally, so as to return to the weight I'd enjoyed in my early thirties. (Actually, I never *enjoyed* that or any other weight. I always thought I was fat even when I wasn't, because "fat," to most full-bodied young women in America, means "subpar," and that's how most of us feel in our heart of hearts as we emerge from adolescence.)

The pasta dinner and many more like it were courtesy of my friend and neighbor Marie, who stayed on an AeroBed in my guest room while her apartment was being renovated. She brought along her two cats to add to my own two cats and a parrot, so it was like an extended slumber party, only with hairballs.

"Would you like me to pay rent?" she asked. I was tempted—free cash!—but I didn't feel right taking money.

"How about if you make the coffee?" Marie is Cuban and learned from her mother that if the coffee isn't just so, the day is shot; Marie makes a damn fine cup of coffee. "And maybe you could cook dinner every now and then."

Marie's cooking is not particularly low-cal. It's simply *lower*-cal than what I'd been eating. Beforehand, I'd grab meals on the run or snack mindlessly at my computer. On days when I need to see three movies with only a 20-minute break, the handiest food to grab (or so it always seemed) was a Starbucks coffee and a slab of lemon-iced pound cake. The relative dryness of the cake intensified the coffee-ness of the coffee. Life was good.

MARIE'S SEAFOOD STEW

Marie usually makes this up as she goes along; this is her latest version.

SERVES 4

Olive oil, just enough to coat pan

1 medium yellow onion, chunk-chopped

4 garlic cloves, minced

One large can crushed tomatoes, with liquid

Seasonings: salt and pepper, thyme, oregano, Tabasco or other hot sauce, prepared horseradish, lemon

About 20 black kalamata olives or marinated black olives, pitted, then quartered or sliced

6-ounce bottle clam juice

Dry white wine, about ⅓ bottle

About ½ pound each of three types of fish with different textures—I prefer calamari, sea scallops, and a firm white fish like catfish, but shrimp can be substituted for the scallops, clams for calamari, salmon for catfish.

Four slices olive bread (or other firm-grained bread), toasted

Lemon

Feta cheese (about 4 ounces), crumbled

Parsley or cilantro (Jami hates cilantro, poor thing)

Heat a large saucepan or stockpot (at least 3 quarts) over a medium-high flame. When the pan is warm, add a touch of olive oil.

Add the onion chunks and the garlic. Sauté, stirring to avoid burning, about 5 minutes. When the onions are soft and before the garlic burns, add the crushed tomatoes.

Add the seasonings while the tomatoes heat: add salt and pepper, sprinkle a small amount of thyme and larger amount of oregano, about 6 to

10 drops of Tabasco, about one teaspoon horseradish. When in doubt, use less—as the stew heats, adjust seasonings to taste.

Add the olives.

When the tomatoes start to simmer, add ½ bottle of clam juice. Reduce the heat and partly cover. Simmer for about 30 to 45 minutes in total to reduce tomatoes and blend flavors. As the stew thickens, add the wine, for flavor and to offset the loss of tomato liquid. The final texture should be a hearty soup.

While the stew simmers, prepare the seafood. The calamari should be cleaned and cut into rings. (Jami says don't clean calamari yourself; it's disgusting.) Cut fish into large chunks. If using sea scallops, cut in half.

This is a good time to toast the bread. It doesn't matter if it gets a bit hard before serving, because it's going to sop up the juices.

When the tomato mixture has simmered sufficiently, raise the heat slightly and add the seafood. The order in which it's added should match the different times it takes to cook. Fish needs the longest cooking time, about 7 minutes. Scallops need about 4 minutes. Calamari and shrimp need less than 2 minutes.

Take the stew off the flame as soon as the seafood is firm.

Place a slice of toasted bread at the bottom of each of four soup or pasta bowls. Spoon the stew over the bread, which will soak up the liquid, further thickening the stew after it's served and intensifying the taste.

Finish with fresh ground pepper and a spritz of lemon for freshness.

Place crumbled feta cheese and a bowl of herbs (parsley or cilantro) on the table so diners can garnish the dish to taste.

Much of my weight gain came from not paying attention, from idly picking up a fork when my mind was elsewhere. But Marie and I would kick back and laugh over pasta (usually with vegetable- or tomato-based sauces) and wine, returning the dinner hour to the social realm, where it belonged. Good food deserves your attention and respect. Bad food should have no place in your life except when there's nowhere else to stop along the Interstate. (But don't get Wendy's Mandarin Chicken Salad; it has 700 calories.)

My African gray parrot, Sensei, would mistake our laughter for a sign that the flock was calling, so she chuckled along in our own voices, which made us laugh harder. Mealtimes were fun and relaxed. And I began to lose weight.

Not a lot of weight. But at 230 pounds, you can probably eat one fewer Mallomar and knock off 10 pounds easy.

Easy-ish, anyway. It helps if you go to the gym. But I had a simple little rule: *I would never join another gym.*

I collect gym memberships the way others collect *Star Wars* action figures. I've joined 'em all. I joined and joined. I paid membership fees, took initiation tours, staked out the best lockers (where the fewest passers-by can see you naked), kept gym bags packed and ready

I'd even work out once or twice. Then I'd stop going.

That's the way gyms make money. A huge percentage of sign-ups never return to shed a drop of sweat, so the gyms sell a gazillion memberships on the safe bet there won't be a line for the adductor machine.

The first gym I ever joined was the Paris, a tony health club being built on the Upper West Side when I was just out of college. It offered discounts if you "pre-joined." Judy Collins was one of the first to come on board; I was close behind. After the ribbon-cutting ceremony, I made a few brief appearances, lifted the occasional weight, soothed myself with calorie-dense "health" drinks at the "health" bar, and looked in vain for signs of Judy. Then I stopped going, abruptly.

My fundamental ambivalence about embracing that gym kicked over into the red after an incident that occurred while I was trundling home in my sweats. It was along a stretch of Broadway that at the time was an armpit of a neighborhood (and which today is so pricey I could never hope to live there). A shadowy figure was following me. "Looks like you need a little help there," he said. I'm still not sure what that meant—I needed a support bra? a spotter?—but I increased my pace and zipped my jacket.

"You can't hide them titties," he taunted.

I ducked into a macrobiotic diner to stop the sleazeball from following me home and leaving a slime trail, like snails do, along Broadway. Did Judy Collins have to put up with this?

The exercise I'd been so proud of was curdling into something sordid. My body, not for the first time, was a source of shame.

When I got home, I did what I always did when I felt powerless, frightened, and enraged—I ate. That'll show 'em! I ate a frozen cheesecake straight from the freezer, impatiently flaking off pieces in a swirl around its frosty edges because I couldn't wait for it to thaw, circling in on its ice-

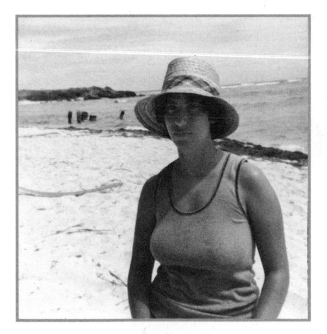

Couldn't hide 'em.

hard center like a vulture, chewing angrily, smothering my rage in food. Cheesecake becomes a paste in the mouth, muffling the inner scream. I couldn't think of any other way to deal. I couldn't become a heroin addict because I'm a needlephobe. Exercise was out; *I can't hide them titties.*

I never went back to the Paris. It doesn't take all that much to leak the air out of those self-improvement tires, and my idiot stalker seemed excuse enough to stall an exercise routine that hadn't really taken hold in the first place.

Different song, same refrain for subsequent gyms. I'd start strong, gamely taking step aerobics or swimming laps, then succumb to feeling subhuman because I didn't look perfect in Lycra and wasn't able to do a split like the gazelles in the locker room. I was always the one who didn't know how to "grapevine." Actually, I *do* know how to grapevine, but I'm dyslexic, so telling me in the heat of a class to step to the right is pointless.

A laminated health-club membership pass makes a good coaster for a big martini.

No more gyms. Marie should've known that. But one day when I was in a foul mood, Marie loomed over me as I was busy self-destructing on the sofa. "Come with me to my gym," she commanded.

"No!" I snarled.

"Why not?"

"Because!" I retorted, displaying further evidence of my finely honed Ivy League education.

Marie continued to stand there, hands on hips. She gave me The Nose, her patented crinkle of nasal displeasure.

This made me furious. *What does she know about anything?* I was about to launch into a tirade against Marie's bossy ways and how her cats drool when they sleep when I suddenly caught a glimpse of how ridiculous I was being. Here was a friend holding out a helping hand; why was I not taking it?

"Okay, *but I'm only gonna swim!*" I threatened.

Swimming doesn't burn many calories and doesn't build much muscle, Olympic athletes aside. I wasn't going to the gym for "exercise"—I wouldn't give them the satisfaction!—I was just doing a few idle laps because I happen to love being in the water. I'd just read the Scott Berg biography of Katharine Hepburn, who took a swim most days of her life, even in the rain. I thought it'd be nice if the same could be said of me: *She swam.* I wouldn't want it to be the *only* thing said of me, but it could go right under "Loved gadgets."

I swam. It was delicious.

"Wait up, Marie!" I called, cheeks bright, eyes sparkling. I needed to stop by the manager's office and sign up for two years at the New York Health & Racquet Club.

I planned only to swim, nothing more—no aerobics, no weights, no pressure (the *Daily News* column was still months away). My immersion into gym culture came slowly, tentatively. I'd arrive for a swim and wonder if I should try a couple of minutes on the elliptical machine—I mean, as long as I was there. Pretty soon, I had a contract with Iva Popovicova, a gorgeous East European personal trainer, and I was spending more time on the treadmill than in the pool. I *wanted* to work out. My body craved it. The days I couldn't go I felt sluggish and disappointed.

I'd never approached a health-club membership from such a laid-back, no-expectations direction. That's because I'd never calibrated my gym habits to what makes me tick: *I don't like being told what to do.*

When I was sixteen, I delayed a high-school concert when the principal told me I couldn't wear a hat while accompanying the choir on the piano. The choir couldn't sing the "Hallelujah Chorus" without me, but I wasn't going to play a single left-hand octave without my floppy blue denim hat.

Had the principal pointed out how ugly the hat was, he might have appealed to my vanity. But he claimed I couldn't wear it because it was "against the rules." *What rules?* The only rule on the books was that we couldn't wear black armbands, a holdover from the era of the Vietnam War.

I stood fast. I argued. I won. I performed at the assembly with my stupid denim hat on.

So while it's true that I like to leap headfirst, do the Weekend Warrior thing, join a gym on a whim and knock myself senseless the first day (and never return), what drives me hardest is my aversion to authority. Nobody's the boss o' me! What I'd needed all along was to embrace exercise at my own pace and on my own terms, a little at a time, playing to my actual strengths instead of to what I thought *ought* to be my strengths. This actually went against everything I believed about myself—that I was wildly impulsive, impetuous, madcap. I had to push past my superficial dream of myself to the sometimes disappointing reality.

It turns out I'm not madcap. I'm not a wild, free spirit who plunges in, a silver flash of gossamer. I'm methodical and oppositional.

By approaching the new gym membership in a way that truly suited my personality, I was able to stick with it and gradually make it mine. For the past few years, I've gone to that same gym and its affiliates up to five times a week. I don't always like the teachers, but no one incident can send me away. I've tried their special programs in Muay Thai kickboxing and Pilates. I go alone or I meet my friend Diane Stefani there for body sculpt. Marie and I do the elliptical together; she claims her heart rate is lower when she exercises with a friend. Helene drops off her toddlers with the babysitting service and we run on the treadmill. I'm a junkie for spin class as long as Pablo Toribio is teaching it; Pablo was named best indoor group cycling instructor in *New York* magazine, but more important, he looks good in Lycra shorts and says inspirational things like, *"Jami's in the house!"*

I am, indeed, *in the house*. But at first, during the initial 10 pounds, I was able to manage only an occasional leisurely 20-minute swim and a few semihealthful meals.

Oh, and one small behavioral change.

"No more ice cream," suggested Stephen Josephson, a behaviorist I consulted out of curiosity to see what other tweaks and adjustments were within grasp. "Unless it's low-fat. Either have none at all, or low-fat. The choice is yours."

You can guess which door I chose.

Before Marie moved in for what stretched to six months, I'd gotten into the gluey habit of eating a pint of ice cream nearly every night. I didn't even pretend to put it in a bowl. Godiva makes a particularly enticing vanilla with chocolate-covered caramel hearts embedded like precious stones.

Binge eaters don't appreciate an audience, so when Marie was around I was unable to fall into a deep ice-cream trance. But I could get near enough to the experience by switching to low-fat frozen yogurt, which is moderately lower in calories. For Marie's sake I made a pretense of eating it from a bowl like a human being. Even if I polished off the whole pint, I was still cutting my former ice-cream intake by 500 calories a day. And Marie, bless her heart, mistakes "low-fat frozen yogurt" for a health food, so she'd smile benignly as I spooned it up, whereas if she'd caught me diving into a tub of Godiva she'd have given me The Nose.

After three weeks of fiddling with my quotient of frozen delights, I downsized again—this time from fat-free frozen yogurt to sorbet. A pint of sorbet is 400 calories, whereas a pint of full-fat ice cream can run you 1500. (I am sorry to report that gelato is not sorbet. Read the fine print.)

Further down the road, I took a meeting with the Nutrition Twins, Lyssie Lakatos and Tammy Lakatos Shames, lissome blond health consultants and gigglers and the authors of *Fire Up Your Metabolism*. If you need to tell them apart, Lyssie is 17 minutes older.

"We used to eat doughnuts for breakfast!" said Lyssie, or maybe it was Tammy. "But when we were eighteen we realized some foods made us feel bad, and we made the association between what we ate and how we performed athletically."

The Twins frightened me the first time we met by whipping out from their closet, like a Halloween prop, a "pound of fat"—a visual aid made of a squishy, fleshy synthetic material. The pinkish blob is the size and weight of, yes, a pound of fat. "You've lost so many of these!" they chortled. "Think of that!" I did, in nightmare after nightmare.

"A pound of muscle looks like a small pager, hard and compact, while a pound of fat looks like this"—they waved the grotesque thing—"a blob of cottage cheese in the bottom of a stocking, loose and unshapely, and double the size of the pager."

Good to know.

I went to them for help with portion control. "How do you handle leftovers?" asked Tammy, or maybe it was Lyssie.

Leftovers weren't a problem. As we overeaters like to say, "Leftovers? What are leftovers?"

★ Thanksgiving Triage

The Nutrition Twins on how to handle holiday leftovers:

Stuffing: "Lower the calories by stirring in several cups of steamed vegetables and tossing in a couple of tablespoons of sunflower seeds for a satiating combo of fiber, extra vitamins, and protein."

Pumpkin pie: "Get rid of the fatty crust and put the filling in small bowls like a pudding. Top with fat-free Reddi-wip."

Potatoes and yams: "Make them into a purée to spread on your bread, rather than using butter."

Cranberry sauce: "Use as a salad dressing."

The Twins' book has solid information, despite chapter titles showing they're as fond of alliteration as some people are of potato chips; you can read about why you should never skip a meal in Chapter 7, "Missing Meals: Misdemeanor or Manslaughter?"

The Twins suggested I switch my nightly sorbet ritual to a package of sugar-free Jell-O with fat-free Reddi-wip. Total calories: 50. That would slice *1450 calories* off my former daily intake without changing anything else while providing a semblance of the sweet and creamy mouthfeel of ice cream.

Okay, you're recoiling in horror. I realize that Jell-O is a poor substitute for caramel-studded ice cream. But remember, this shift was gradual, and that's the point: I was eased into new eating habits, not pushed off the diet cliff. By the time I got to sugar-free Jell-O I had long since lost the taste for full-fat ice cream, which now seemed unpleasantly thick and slimy. My friend Amanda, the Exercise Nazi, had always claimed that if you cut down on fat and grease long enough you lose your taste for it. I never believed her . . . until now.

You can't go around thinking it's a choice in life between Godiva or Jell-O, satiety or deprivation, the lady or the tiger. Think instead, what do I get out of this one particular food habit (sweetness, creaminess, a sense of indulgence, a treat before bed), and how can I replicate that through inventive substitution?

Going from ice cream to low-fat frozen yogurt to sugar-free Jell-O was my own personal methadone program. It took two months of concerted effort to change that one food addiction. In the throes of a diet mentality, two months would be an eternity, and the typical all-or-nothing dieter would never put in that kind of time. If they don't see fat fall from their hips within minutes of tearing the plastic membrane off a container of low-fat cottage cheese, they're outta there.

But I hung in, losing surely, if nearly imperceptibly, one dainty pound a week or less.

It was a beautiful thing.

20 POUNDS:
THE SHOP AROUND
THE CORNER

December 28, 1964: Today Diane sneaked out to buy two wafers (she gave me one, and I have to pay her back 5 cents) and Sour Tarts. (I'll pay her back for that too. She just gave me a little, though.)

Give me your money."

Diane, two and a half years older, had cornered me in our shared bedroom and was demanding a cut of my 50-cent allowance.

Diane wasn't a bully in the usual sense, not like the bullies at school who stole my lunch money and made me watch them buy pizza with it. (Food and humiliation, forever joined at the hip.) My sister was more of an intellectual bully. She had big plans for my allowance, plans that would benefit me, like an investment in an African diamond mine. "I'll buy us two red-fur rabbit's feet," she explained.

Who knows why we needed red rabbit's feet? Diane made everything sound reasonable, including the time she traded me a piece of string for my beautiful Catherine doll. *A ratty piece of string.* Diane could talk me into anything.

She smuggled my two quarters to the corner candy store like a double agent lurking behind enemy lines. She made it back in one piece and gave me my rabbit's foot.

But not my change.

What could I do? Complain to Mom and see that rabbit's foot go down the rabbit hole of the incinerator room? During one of her Richter-scale furies, Mom had disappeared my collection of *Mad* magazines, Sandinista-style. A rabbit's foot in her possession didn't stand a chance.

I named the rabbit's foot Lucky after the unlucky animal to which it had once been attached. The charm afforded little pleasure. Nevertheless, Diane taught me a valuable skill set that day: sneaking around the corner to the candy store on Northern Boulevard.

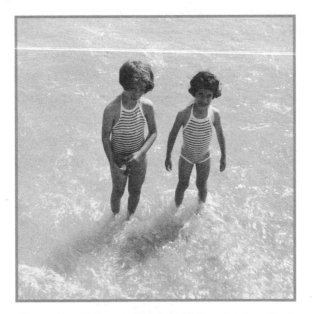

Sister swimsuits for me (right) and Diane, Brighton Beach.
(Photo by Sam Bernard)

Pretty soon, I cut out the middleman. No more Diane to cheat me of my change, to buy treats with my money and repay me less than my fair quota of Sour Tarts. I discovered I could buy anything I wanted—nothing cost more than a nickel in those days—egg creams, licorice whips, powdered-sugar Pixy Stix, chalky Chocolate Babies. I didn't even like some of those candies, but taste wasn't as important as fun. Candy dots are merely hardened lumps of colored sugar, but prying them off the paper strip with your teeth was engrossing. They never came off clean; there were always bits of paper still attached that got balled up in your mouth after the sugar melted. That in itself was an adventure.

Seeking fun from your food isn't just for kids. How else to explain elusive escargots plucked from whorled shells with surgically precise utensils? Or tearing sticky-saucy shreds of meat from barbecued ribs? Or harvesting the glistening ruby eggs from a pomegranate? The pleasures of food go far beyond taste, let alone its value as fuel for the body. Food is sensuous entertainment for all ages.

Sneaking candy was a thrilling adventure, my little secret. So what if it was quasi-sordid? It was something of my own, away from prying eyes, something—I see this now in retrospect—to do with my body that no one was controlling or inspecting or analyzing.

I'd duck around the corner to eat my stash, hunched furtively near the redbrick side of the corner candy store or pretending to search for the family car in the parking lot behind the playground. The crispy chocolate mounds of the 100 Grand bar came two to a package, a bonus! Even better were M&M's or Rolos, because you could hide them in your pocket and fish out a few at a time as if surprised to find them there, a combination of crunchy and chewy. I'd eat them hastily, delirious with pleasure, trembling with guilt.

There's nothing wrong with adoring the sybaritic pleasures of texture, taste, aroma. But my secretive behavior around certain foods was emanating from a bad place. I wanted, needed. Something was missing, even from the earliest age. My yearning for something of my own—something delicious, secret, and unshared—plus the rush that came from disobeying my parents, overcame the shame that quickly attached itself to the act of consuming candy. I was a bad girl. I was spending allowance money that doubtless should have been earmarked for a Mother's Day gift. I was shrouded in self-loathing.

I began to do it more often.

> *December 30, 1964:* Nancy's birthday [Nancy was one of Diane's dolls] was supposed to be on Christmas, but we forgot the party so on New Years we'll take French pastries, stuff them in our pockets, and when Mom is out going around at night we'll give them to our dolls.

Dolls, my ass.

Sneaking food became natural, as integral to childhood as hopscotch. Diane and I were hollow and aching, a gnawing condition fostered in part by the ancestral sense of deprivation our parents brought along from their own childhoods. The Depression and World War II defined my parents' generation solely, I think, so they could say things like "Poverty? *You don't know poverty!*" or "Vietnam? That's *nothing!*" My family's predisposition for negativity and alarm (*"You'll catch pneumonia!"*) was compounded by the certainty that disaster was imminent—Daddy would lose his job. The Nazis would return to power. (*"And they'll find you,"* warned my mother darkly after I changed my religion at thirteen.)

Faded pictures of my father show that it's not as if he had nothing to eat in his youth. Nevertheless, he grew up to clip and hoard coupons like war rations. He cleaned out the local Safeway during its 2-for-1 sales

Wednesday, January 1, 1964

1st day – 365 days follow

Dear Anne,
I had a party.
I had ddnuts,
chease flavered
fish crackers,
Pizza flafered fish crakk-
-rs, Hershy m and
m's, asorted candy,
and Po-ta-to
chips. We danced
to the record
kiss me kate
and I got growing
pains. I had the
party at 7:30
in the evenig.
Yesterday I wacthd
Kiss Me Kate. I am
planning to see it again.

on canned pineapple; we found his stash in the recesses of the pantry after his death.

I learned about hoarding—both food and material things—at the knees of people who thought it immoral to discard anything (*"You never know . . ."*). At least they stopped short of making one of those giant balls from old rubber bands, or collapsing beneath the weight of yellowed newspapers like the Collyer brothers. Remember, they had no use for my *Mad* magazines, so they were willing to make the occasional exception.

I enjoyed a fairly benign upbringing in blue-collar Queens—Daddy worked on the overnight mail trains, Mom was a part-time secretary, Diane and I went to public schools and spent summers in the Poconos. We had a car and a hamster and, eventually, a dishwasher and (wow!) a reel-to-reel tape recorder.

Yet I grew up deprived. Or it felt that way. The bottomless pit that I gradually mistook for hunger had only tangentially to do with nutrition. Early on, food and despair merged in my mind into one big ball of indigestible crud.

> *January 1, 1964:* I had a party. I had donuts, cheese flavored fish crackers, pizza flavored fish crackers, Hershey M&Ms, assorted candy, and potato chips. We danced to the record Kiss Me Kate.
>
> *December 31, 1964:* Mommy set out raisins, nuts, round pretzels, and potato chips. We had a lot. We watched Jonny Quest, Daniel Boone, Perry Mason and Bewitched.

Ah, my diaries. I saved them all except for the one about shaking hands with astronaut John Glenn. The diaries detail my ruses for staying home from school (nosebleed, "sic" feeling, "temperture") and the roll call of my toys (the gummy plastic cavemen from outer space; Pixie the bone-china horse with her foals Dixie and Pixacita; and the Evil Uncle, a plastic "workman" whose yellow hardhat unscrewed to reveal within his hollow, liver-colored trunk a dose of noxious iron supplement for my anemia). The diaries are packed with descriptions of what we watched on TV, down to changes in the seasonal lineup. From December 24, 1964:

> Jonny Quest and Daniel Boone from Friday were changed to Thursday when the Munsters were on. The Flintstones from Thursday was changed to Friday. The Addams Family and The Farmer's Daughter stayed the same time on Friday.

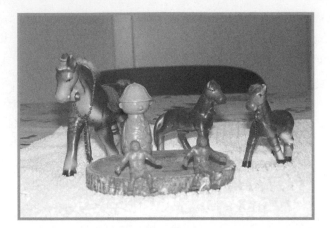

The childhood toys, rescued from the incinerator room.

Not exactly wisdom for the ages, whereas other entries contained deep, deep thoughts:

> *January 13, 1968:* It seems impossible that space doesn't end. It must have an end. But it doesn't. How can it go on forever? I wish we weren't poor.
>
> *January 22, 1968:* If you really want to know how I feel, you have to read my mind, which wouldn't be pleasant for me. . . . There are lots of things about heart transplants in the news these days. Nice step in medical progress. But I'm only interested in vast space, where no one is unhappy. And yet, one is.

And, under the rubric of "You never know," from April 27, 1968:

> I have been practicing piano with my eyes closed lately. In case I go blind.

Also in the diaries are the seeds of bad eating habits. It didn't seem to matter in those days if I ate badly, because I was skinny and so active that my grandmother was always yelling for me to stop running and sit still. If she could have had me cryogenically frozen, I think she would have. But as I grew less active in early adulthood—a posthumous triumph of my grandmother's hectoring—the calories in/calories out equation began to shift.

> *March 14, 1964:* Today we were getting ready for Diane's party. We went to 500 different stores for candy. At one store we paid four dollars for candy!
>
> *March 15, 1964* (a specil day): Today's Diane's birthday. We went to see Cinerama. It was all red inside. It was a three-demenchenel picture. After, I had an oversized egg sandwich that was popping out all over the place.
>
> *January 16, 1965:* Today I had Chicken Delight and it was delicious. They give you napkins, cranberry sause, mints and salt!

The point of any holiday, excursion, or gathering was the food. Only the wonders of a "three-demenchenel picture" could tear me from the high point of the day: A Vesuvius of a sandwich. The Chicken Delight entry is evidence I was already being seduced by food and its trappings, my head turned by the least little extra—imagine, free napkins! free salt!

When an early McDonald's franchise opened on Astoria Boulevard, it was a big deal. I had my Sweet 16 there. Today a Big Mac is as common as toenails, but at the beginning it was a futuristic novelty like the Belgian waffles at the Belgian Pavilion at the 1964 World's Fair in Queens, or the

Sloppy Joes made in what the fair billed as the first microwave oven. (Between stops for snacks, there was always the fair's memorable Festival of Gas or the House of Good Taste.)

I was in awe of exotic food—exotic being anything that wasn't in my mother's modest revolving menu.

> *Jan. 17, 1965:* Today I watched The Wizard of Oz. Mommy made her own horrible chicken with skin.

I undervalued food, I overvalued it. I hated Hamburger Helper, which tasted like a chemical bath, yet I wolfed it down whenever it was available; *you never know . . .*

Bad habits from childhood get embedded in your skin like growth rings on a tree. I'd been losing weight on my 100-pound plan at the approximate rate of a pound a week when I found myself cutting into the cherry pie that was meant for the next day's Thanksgiving dinner. As the knife hovered over the pie, a little voice screamed: *"You're stealing the crutches of Tiny Tim!"*

Imagine, taking Thanksgiving food from my own family. The shame! The moral turpitude! The . . . *sweet, sticky cherry glop on a flaky, chewy crust!* I forked it up with one hand while rinsing an air-conditioner filter with the other. Some would call that self-punishment, or at least ambivalence; I call it multitasking.

I'm not a serious binge eater, the

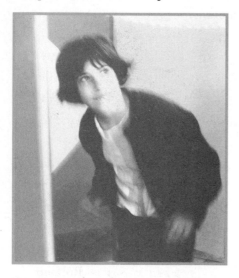

Me, emerging from the Continental Circus at the 1964 World's Fair. The Belgian waffles are all I remember. *(Photo by Sam Bernard)*

kind who can consume a frightening 10,000 calories in a sitting. My relationship with food is the kind that's usually referred to as disordered eating, the garden variety. Half a cherry pie is nothing, at least when compared with a major-league binge. Still, it disturbed me. With that pie in my crosshairs, I rationalized that I'd already logged an hour and a half at the gym that morning. But that kind of calorie bargaining is nonsense. What's destructive beyond the calories is the habit itself. Binge behavior literally feeds on itself, stoking the flame of food desire. Yet I continued to believe I could have "just a little," like an alcoholic in denial who fills a pilsner glass three-quarters full with whiskey and counts it as one drink.

The fact that I had already lost weight ensured lifetime inoculation against relapse, no? I kept messing with the rules, even though the rules were simple and obvious:

- Grilled before fried.
- Whole-grain over white.
- No cherry pies in the house overnight.

There are degrees of food illness. Howard Rankin, a psychologist specializing in weight disorders, told me of a clinic patient who crept into the kitchen one night to drink 19 pints of milk. I've never eaten out of the garbage, although George Costanza did on *Seinfeld*. I don't raid the refrigerator in the middle of the night. I'm not *sloppy*-fat.

The biggest binge Rankin knew of involved 75,000 calories. To consume that amount, you'd have to eat the equivalent of 25 Caramel Kreme Crunch doughnuts from Krispy Kreme (8,750 calories), four Double-Doubles at In-N-Out Burger (1,770), eight slices of Sausage Lover's stuffed-crust pizza from Pizza Hut (3,440), 15 beef Chalupa Supremes from Taco Bell (5,850), 70 scoops of Rocky Road from Baskin-Robbins (20,300), 100 Extra Crispy drumsticks from KFC (16,000), five platters of Kung Pao Chicken at P.F. Chang's (6,150), three Mango-A-Go-Go smoothies from Jamba Juice (990), seven large Moo Malts from TCBY (10,920), four California sushi rolls (830), and one Diet Coke.

So I'm not up there in the big-time pathology leagues with my half a cherry pie. I'm an overeater and a food sneaker, but I'm not sloppy-fat. *I'm not sloppy-fat.*

★ Ingredients of a Binge

Overeating or cleaning your plate is common. A binge is a whole other animal. Psychologist Howard Rankin says there are three things that make a binge a binge: volume, mindlessness, and shame.

The volume has to be excessive, abnormal, and consumed relatively quickly. Mindlessness is where you don't think about what you're eating to the point where you might not even taste it. Shame is both cause and effect of a binge.

According to Rankin, a binge entails all three elements. That all-American pastime the hotdog-eating contest involves volume, but contestants are mindful (they're counting the wieners) and feel no shame (they get applause). Likewise, overindulging at a party isn't a binge—there's volume and mindlessness, but it's a perfectly acceptable misbehavior within a particular social setting.

Rankin calls binge behavior a "disorder of the soul," a response to a feeling of emptiness and an attempt to stuff back or numb feelings of anger, loneliness, frustration, boredom, and depression. "Whenever you use a substance—whether it's drink or cigarettes or food—to manage your emotions, you'll do it compulsively," he says. "Effectively, it becomes a drug, and then this behavior develops a life of its own."

Marie found out the hard way about my food-bandito side when she was staying with me. I'd hear the dreaded sound of the freezer door opening. Some rummaging. Then silence. "What happened to my frozen yogurt?" she'd call upstairs in a level voice, still giving me the benefit of the doubt as if I might throw some light on how a burglar broke in during the night with a bowl and spoon.

"I finished it," I'd reply, nonchalant, as if I'd actually done her a favor, like doing her hand wash or bundling her recyclables.

"You ate my frozen yogurt?" she'd scream. "It was *mine!*"

I threw the blame back on her, my defensiveness ratcheted up by guilt. "*It's your fault.* You know you can't leave me alone in the house with something like that. I can't be responsible for my actions!"

Marie was disgusted, insulted, unnerved. Although she'd lost 35 pounds on Weight Watchers (and has since lost much more), she's one of those rare birds who doesn't really have an eating problem. Once she realized her weight had crept up, she took action, lost the weight precisely on schedule, and never looked back.

I would hate her except she's my friend.

Marie is one of the few females I know who doesn't "get" eating problems. She insists she does. But she doesn't. She's the kind who says, "Just eat less," and means it.

Dieting the KFC Way

If you're trying to lose weight, you shouldn't be anywhere near a KFC. But let's say your kidnapper forced you to go in and order a bucket. Keep in mind: One measly Original Recipe chicken breast is 380 calories. Extra Crispy is 460.

Then there's my friend JoAnne, a reformed food stealer. In her twenties, during a summer share on the Jersey shore, she ate all the frosting off her roommate's birthday cake the night before the celebration. "Did I ever tell you about the time I ate Hope the dancer's cake?" she asked in a recent e-mail. "Squatting in front of the fridge and leaving these disgusting finger marks . . . it's too embarrassing to even continue."

JoAnne used her finger to swirl a little frosting off—who would notice? Then she evened it out and tried another spot. Come morning, Hope the dancer found a naked, desiccated cake, and, like the proverbial cheating husband, JoAnne felt her only recourse was to deny, deny, deny.

JoAnne is still a snacker, a chewer, a muncher. But she's been on the Weight Watchers wagon for most of her adult life, continuing to count points, never going wild. She'll wail over the phone about those last, stubborn three pounds while the sounds of chomping and slurping are amplified through the receiver. "But I *am* exercising! I *stopped* with the bagels!" she'll insist, sentences muffled by juicy swallowing sounds.

I doubt she's gone on a binge since her twenties, when she lost a lot of grief weight (her father died of a sudden heart attack when she was away at college). She has kept it off ever since. Weight Watchers got its claws into her early and she counts points excitedly, like a kid identifying every fire engine and front-loader in sight. She'll pull a box of matchstick pretzels from her desk as if displaying a rare coin and announce, "Only two points! Can you believe it?"

One time in a Japanese restaurant she ordered the safest thing from a calorie point of view, sashimi—raw fish, rice on the side. "How many points d'ya think?" she asked, gesturing with chopsticks toward the inviting slabs of ruby tuna and plump yellowtail.

Sushi chefs take pride in presentation. Dewy undulations of fish are arranged just so around a bundle of wasabi and flower-petal slices of ginger. They craft your dinner to look like living art. So I wanted to commit hara-kiri when JoAnne scooped up her sashimi in one hand—all that uncooked and therefore prone-to-bacteria fish in her germ-laden palm—and hefted it up and down like she's the scales of justice. Waiter, check please!

But she's a changed woman. I'd trust her with my life, maybe even my baked goods.

30 POUNDS:
MY BODY, MYSELF

The driver who paused on Junction Boulevard to give me a lift stared fixedly at my fourteen-year-old, jeans-clad crotch as I climbed into his truck. This, in my experience, was typical, therefore normal.

I was hitchhiking after school to visit my friend Linda in Rego Park, two miles away. I usually biked there, but my father had recently crashed the family bike on Roosevelt Avenue while trying to ride it to his night job. Daddy wound up with a steel implant in his femur; the bike wasn't so lucky.

Hitchhiking wasn't wise, then as now, but I think it was a lot safer then. Getting a lift was never a problem—that was an accepted, unremarkable fact of life for any adolescent girl whose breasts had ripened from grapes to grapefruits overnight.

Breast buds were bursting like popcorn beneath the blouses of girls as young as eleven, but for a long time, it looked like I'd never get a bosom at all. All was quiescent on my smooth, boyish chest until the waning weeks of my twelfth year, when twin Mount St. Helens erupted there, much to the hand-wringing consternation of my parents. My first training bra must've worked, because I didn't need training for long.

Thereafter, drivers, cops, service personnel, even my male schoolteachers treated me like royalty. My most fervent childhood dreams came true: I was indeed the center of the universe, at least wherever there was a grown man behind a counter or steering wheel or in a booth or calling the shots. At supermarkets, box offices, and pizza parlors, of course. At the Wollman Rink in Central Park, where I went three times a week with my best friend Andrea and my babysitting money. Whenever I babysat for Brenda's three kids, the man Brenda was dating was eager to drive me home; he'd have me sit on his lap and steer the car through the parking lot. Men gave me discounts and freebies. They lingered when putting change in my hand so they could stroke my palm meaningfully or scratch out a Helen Keller–like message there with their fingertips. They said ridiculous things; one Wollman Rink guard had me take off my glasses to better see the color of my eyes, then crossed himself and said, "America the Beautiful."

Was I beautiful? Not especially. I'm nice-looking, not gorgeous. I have a nice smile. But the phenomenal burst of attention I received in adolescence was all about my body, specifically my breasts. The Wollman guard wouldn't have crossed himself in ecstasy if I hadn't begun to resemble a junior Chesty Morgan.

I didn't plan it that way, didn't do it on purpose. I didn't wear low-cut, transparent blouses or makeup or anything remotely provocative—my standard uniform into my thirties was jeans and a T-shirt; I hardly owned anything else—yet men on the street responded as if I had sashayed past with a feather boa and stiletto heels. They routinely mistook my body for me and vice versa, leading to a lifetime of trouble and confusion.

And when I sneezed, forget it. I don't know what physiological forces to blame, but when I sneeze I get goosebumps, and two of those strategic goosebumps made me look like a refugee from the porn industry. My nipples would harden and poke through my bra, even sports bras. They could have pierced armor. With every *achoo,* my nipples sent out emergency alert signals that only horny men could see, the equivalent of high-pitched whistles for dogs.

These men assumed it was their manly presence that made my nipples snap to attention. Actually, I had hay fever. Their yearning for me was born in the crucible of my sinus.

A stranger stopped me in the parking lot of the Kentucky Fried Chicken—I was cutting through on the way to eighth grade, thank you very much—to ask whether I was a "working girl." I wasn't familiar with the expression, but I understood by his tone it was a reference to prostitution.

No, I said, confused but polite.

Well then, would I be willing to give him a call when I changed my mind?

Sure, I said.

Sure? I've spent a lifetime not being able to say no for fear of hurting someone's feelings. Men who think that no means yes don't know the real deal: More often, yes means no. Which country is it where shaking the head means yes and nodding means no? I must visit sometime.

Later that day—same boulevard, different cross street—another intrusive stranger informed me that I was "a thoroughbred," which my parents later insisted was a compliment I should be proud of. I mean, a thoroughbred! Not a nag or a brood mare, you know!

I tried—*really tried*—to take these remarks as compliments. But I was furious. These men made me feel that my lissome, curvy body was a thing of lewdness and shame. My ripe adolescent form attracted men who murmured unmistakable come-ons in foreign tongues. My innocent body perked up the homeless and intrigued briefcase-toting businessmen. They leered and whispered, catcalled and made animal sounds. They jangled their keys as if I were a cat attuned to the sound of a can opener on a tin of Friskies. Their attempts to intimidate me into meeting their laser stares made me feel hunted and controlled. My body didn't belong to me, it was in the public domain: *Ka-ching! Looka them titties!*

Only large-breasted women seem to know what I'm talking about. I've yet to find a smaller-busted woman who understands or even *believes* me when I describe what it was like to grow up hounded about my boobs, not just by perverts but by perfectly normal-looking men who unashamedly glued their eyes chest-high. Often I'd be talking with men who stared so fixedly at my chest I had to clap my hands in the air and bark, *"I'm up here!"*

If it had happened only a few times, fine. But this was constant, cease-less, a Chinese water torture of unwanted sexual attention from the day those mounds sprang to life until my mid-thirties, when I purposely sub-sumed them under a bodysuit of adipose tissue. *Stop staring at me, ass-holes!*

So hitchhiking in adolescence was a breeze. I knew I'd get a lift the minute I put my thumb out. Men honked and slowed even when I *didn't* put my thumb out. The only surprise about this particular guy on Junc-tion Boulevard was that he was staring at my crotch, not my boobs; I guess all men have their favorite parts. This one sported the same swollen-lidded, goofy-glazed look they'd all get, like volunteers at a hypnotist's show who soon find themselves barking on all fours.

So this man picked me up and leered all the way to Linda's. I pretended as usual not to notice; heaven forbid I make any of these fellows uncom-fortable or hurt their feelings. He asked me dumb questions all the way to Rego Park, and I answered politely because . . . I didn't know I had any choice. No matter what message my body seemed to send, I was only fourteen. The driver was an *adult,* and it was unthinkable that I, a *child,* could elect not to answer him or tell him to keep his eyes on the road.

Yes, yes, I know that kids are different these days, they grow up so fast.

But I'd only recently realized that I was allowed to ride up front with the driver instead of taking the traditional child's place in the back seat.

Men looked at me and saw the body of a woman. But I was a kid, a virgin, a "good girl" despite my smart mouth and C cup.

Since no one had thought to tell me otherwise, I learned and accepted that it was my lot to suffer implied sexual pressure at all times from men no matter where I went, in return for the everyday things I was still too powerless or penniless to get for myself. If it hadn't been the guy in the truck on Junction, it would have been an overly solicitous bus driver (if I'd had the bus fare, which I didn't, because all my babysitting money went toward ice skating). Or it would have been a handyman or a friend's father. Even teachers overstepped their bounds, and in hindsight it makes me furious—like the married writing teacher who tongue-kissed me at fifteen after telling me how talented I was. (I couldn't say no—he might take back the compliment!) The air around me was humid and foul with the lust of authority figures who should've protected me from exactly this kind of sexual pressure. They thought I was fair game because they presumed, or wished, that my body said so.

When I got out of the truck, the driver pointed to my crotch and said, "Take care of that, li'l lady." Meaning, I presume, something more intimate than remembering to schedule an annual Pap smear.

"*Oh, I will!*" I promised, so earnestly I could puke. My eyes shimmered, as if moist with tears at his tender concern. Yes, I will take care of "that," I *will*, I'll offer it only strategically to a select few, as it is my one true prize, sir.

My eyes weren't shining because I thought he cared or because I'd mistaken his sleazy interest for something more profound, or even because I was trying to be the worldly woman he might have thought I was. They glistened because *I felt beholden to him for the goddamn lift* and was doing my best to act suitably grateful. Otherwise, who knows, maybe he'd take it away from me, force me back in the truck and drive me back to Square

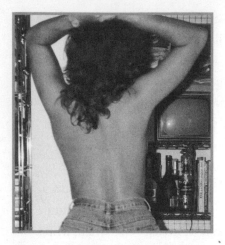

Friends don't let friends drink and let their boyfriends take "fun" pictures.

One, where I'd have to thumb another lift and act suitably grateful all over again.

I wasn't a working girl, no, but I was trading away the sense of ownership of my body for the price of carfare.

Right after college—and then I'll drop the subject, I promise—I lived in an off-brand, largely Hispanic neighborhood full of burned-out lots where they sold Christmas trees in winter and drugs the rest of the year. I bounced along these semi-mean streets while male passersby acted like a Greek chorus, commenting on my every physical feature. When they sensed I wasn't receptive, their admiration turned to fury and they hurled epithets—*dyke!*—so that on my approach it was all hip-thrusting come-ons, and as I moved beyond them it turned to harsh invective, creating a kind of sexual Doppler effect I experienced anytime I set foot out the door.

I talked back at first: *"Fuck you!"* I screamed in a howl of early eighties feminist rage. It only inflamed them. The best remedy was to remain silent and fix my gaze in the middle distance as if I hadn't noticed them blocking my path or heard them detailing what they'd do to me in bed, one man's fantasy barely out of hearing range before the guy on the next stoop started in. They tried to get my attention with bizarre behavior that could come only from some tone-deaf sex manual—*Picking Up Chicks for Dummies*—like sucking their teeth or making undulating mouth motions like babies learning to sound out vowels. The key jangling was my personal favorite for its implicit assumption that women come when they're called, like dogs.

There was power in my denims. It disgusted and thrilled me. I loved my body, knew it was special, proudly wore T-shirts that were form-fitting without being vulgar, pranced and strutted with the glory of youth. But my body seemed to invite shame, and this push-pull over the years gradually distanced me from my physical self. Over here was *me*, over there was my body, roommates barely on speaking terms. No wonder when I overate I had no sense of repercussions; for that I'd have to *own* my body, not just drape clothing on it.

This rift between the ectoplasm that was "me" and the physical presence that was my body had to heal in order for me to lose weight. It didn't happen quickly. It was two years into the weight-loss process when, while taking a swim, it suddenly hit me: *I'm in love with my body again!* It wasn't just because of the weight loss. I'd looked at myself naked in the locker room mirror moments before and noted, serenely and without rancor, that I was still lumpy here and there. Yet I love my body! I'm satisfied with it . . . with *me*. You don't need to look like a model to take pride in your body. You don't have to look great or even good. It's because the simple act of *feeling* your body, being one with it, is what constitutes physical self-love. Knowing it intimately, not judging it aesthetically.

I know so many women with lovely figures who hate their bodies. It's insane. They find fault with discrete body parts as if rejecting paint colors. They say, "Ick, I hate my thighs" in the certainty that the next and only step is to improve those thighs into lovability; firm and reduce them, slenderize and reshape them. *Then* they will love their thighs.

But they won't. There's always another flaw on which to fixate. Disdain for your body is a free-floating disappointment that has nothing to do with . . . *your body*. Those who are tormenting their thighs into presumed acceptability are working on the wrong self-improvement project. Accepting your flaws leads to body love, not the other way around—and acceptance here simply means not passing judgment.

I'm wildly excited about this discovery. You don't have to work yourself to death to achieve perfect arms or pay a plastic surgeon to craft perky breasts. The externals won't change your intrinsic view of yourself. Your time needs to be spent becoming one with yourself.

For some, that means joining a drum circle. Too bad I'm not into that. Simply exercising, paying attention to my body, strengthening it, feeding it properly, luxuriating in my strength, all of that gradually turned "it" into "me." My body, myself! Without realizing it, I'd grown to love me again instead of singling out aspects of myself to love (I'm good with animals!). It's another key to weight loss: The goal isn't for the cerebral part of you to whip the corporal part into shape so it can be trotted out in polite company wearing the perfect little black dress. *The goal is to show yourself respect by treating your body well.* Weight loss, once again, is a happy by-product of healthy living, not an end in itself.

It was a long time coming, this body acceptance. I began by exercising in that angry way people have when they're out of touch with themselves, exercise as punishment or repentance—I'll do one last push-up if it kills me! My body was an embarrassment, something to be dragged along behind me, to apologize for. Exposing my body in public, let alone drawing attention to it, could be mortifying—like that time I destroyed the purple dragon float in the pool of the ultra-trendy Standard Hotel in L.A., a hotel that prides itself on being cool and unusual; there's a glass tank behind the reception desk where an underclad model pretends to read or nap. Without these little touches, the Standard would be, well, *standard.* Having a fat person doing abs crunches in the pool is *sub*-standard. I had to psych myself up just to feel entitled to get into their stupid pool.

After what happened there, I didn't feel entitled to live.

The purple dragon was a segmented float, and it would still be floating if I hadn't jumped on it to do abs crunches like I'd learned in aquasize class. The float ripped apart with a Velcro-like wrenching sound and two purple Bratwurst links drifted apart, accusingly. I tried to herd them into the deep end, containing them like an oil spill. The trendy lunch crowd, most of them Ethan Hawke lookalikes with sprayed-on tans and scripts in lap, were aghast.

I later asked the hotel gardener with studied casualness what happened to the purple dragon. "I had to dispose of it," he said darkly. *"It was mauled."*

"Surely it wasn't mauled?" I asked.

"Mauled," he repeated.

The fat girl had slain the dragon.

There was a rumor that the Standard was getting a starfish float, but I had already packed my bags.

At least I was trying to exercise. It's possible to lose weight solely by cutting calories, but it's hard, and it deprives you of the health benefits of strong bones and powerful lungs. Exercise revs up the metabolism so you can get away with eating more. Exercise makes you glow.

Studies show that people won't use a gym unless it's within four miles of home, a meaningless statistic for Manhattanites. Here, if the gym isn't on your block, in your building, or in your bed, it's not close enough. In any case, the four-mile rule doesn't seem to apply to me. For years I kept a huge, gleaming home gym in my guest room. There was no room for guests; when Marie stayed over she had to shove her AeroBed right up to the base of the pec deck. For a while I used the equipment regularly, but eventually it turned into a museum installation that you regard from a distance so as not to degrade it with oily fingerprints.

It turns out I prefer a workout environment that's a destination. It doesn't live in my home wagging a finger at me. I like the structure of going to a gym, taking a class, showering, moving on.

Still, I hated being the fattest person in the class, sometimes the slowest. It was ages before I was no longer the weakest link. It's not that my progress was unusually slow, more that those classes attract regulars who are just in for a little fitness touch-up. Even now that I'm up to speed, more or less, there are mornings when I'm less than magnanimous; after exhausting myself on a difficult set of maneuvers, I'll look up and see half the women still pumping away, hardly breaking a sweat. *Bitches.*

You don't have to join a gym to get exercise—there are parks to jog in and stairs to climb everywhere, all free. Mall walking will no doubt be an Olympic sport one day. Still, gyms have the edge. They have one and only one purpose: to pick up strangers for casual sex. Okay, two purposes, the second being that they offer a dedicated space for fitness, with all the equipment, resources, and encouragement you need. If you're in a park, you have too many nonexercise options, like sitting on a bench or firing up a hibachi. If you're mall walking with a credit card tucked in your waistband, forget it, the only aerobic workout you'll get is from lugging your packages to the car. But in a gym you're far more likely, as the Nike ads say, to Just Do It.

One caveat, though: If you're new to exercise or think you hate it, *don't take a class at a gym.* I mean it. Shield your eyes and move away from Studio A, where the body-fitness workshop is in progress. Don't chance it or you'll end up frustrated. You'll never go back, your weight-loss program will be in tatters, you'll hate yourself, you'll hate anyone in the class who warms up ostentatiously by doing splits at the barre.

I'm not saying don't join a gym. But it's the rare gym that offers a true beginner class, the kind that introduces you to proper form and where you're not mowed down by a stampede of babes in spandex.

Maybe it's different in the rest of the country. But in New York, gym classes are filled with models, actors, ballerinas, and Broadway hoofers. They're all double-jointed. They share a special intuition about what move comes next. I took one class at a trendy gym overlooking the Hudson River where the instructor used the subtlest of hand gestures, a sort of fitness sign language that takes years of study to interpret. In this silent class—Aerobics for Mimes?—everyone knew what to do and moved through the routine fluidly. Except me, who had to take Intro to Tap Dance twice in order to fulfill my college gym requirement, repeating the class be-cause of that dyslexia. ("Shuffle off to Buffalo to the left! *To the left!*")

The people who go to these classes are *regulars*. They know the drill. Here's a clue: If the class description says it's designed for "all levels," what it really means is "all levels, like Olympic gold, silver, or bronze."

My neighbor Helene once talked me into taking a class in capoeira, a dancelike Brazilian martial art repurposed as fitness routine. I should've been tipped off by the description: "all levels." Plus, Helene took spin classes well into her ninth month of pregnancy, which terrorized the in-structors, and recently she's been training for triathlons. All I can say is, Helene, *you go girl*. But please go without me.

In capoeira, they had us balance awkwardly for what was essentially a one-armed handstand. For "all levels."

It was the beginning of the end for that particular membership; another gym bites the dust.

Classes where you can't keep up make you feel bad. If you *must* en-dure this humiliation, at least pull the teacher aside, introduce your-self, and say you're new and would welcome special instruction on form, technique, and how to mod-ify the exercises for your level. Had I taken that precaution with capoeira, I'm sure they would have figured out something easier for me, like hanging off a cliff by my fingernails.

I didn't take gym classes at New York Health & Racquet Club until

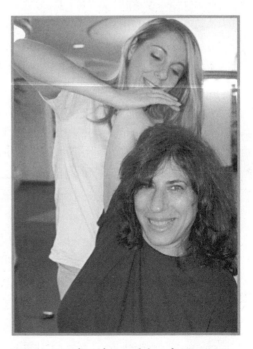

Triceps stretch with Iva *(Photo by Tanya Bra-ganti, courtesy New York* Daily News*)*

I'd worked out one-on-one with Iva Popovicova for several months. Iva's a gorgeous girl from the Czech Republic who doesn't realize there's clothing here in America that's designed to cover the abdomen; I must take her shopping. She seems unaware of her ripe beauty. But she's certainly aware of how men react to her—the ol' googly-eyed thing I remember from adolescence.

It's funny, because they've got her so wrong; she's finishing up her Ph.D. on Eastern European women's political art. All the men can see is long blond hair, taut belly, tantalizing strength; invisible to them is the kind of intellectual discussion that really turns her on.

We ran a picture in the paper of Iva training me, and she was unhappy with how she looked. Like many thin people, however, she doesn't turn her anger inward, stuffing her feelings down with a pile of pasta. Instead—this is so healthy!—she turns the anger outward. I just happened to be standing in the way.

Iva "I'm not mad at you, per se" Popovicova meted out punishment for that photo with heavier weights, more reps, and a jump rope.

"I thought you looked babelicious!" I panted.

"*Jump,*" said Iva, channeling the Communist bureaucrats of her childhood.

Personal trainers are pricey, no question. But it's a worthwhile investment to get at least an introductory session to learn the essentials. Otherwise, you can easily pull or strain something. More likely, you'll expend needless energy on workouts that are counterproductive. I've had plenty of personal training and there's still much to learn. I only recently discovered I've been doing squats all wrong. I wasn't sticking my ass out enough. Only when your ass sticks out so far that it's across the street are you doing it right.

Speaking of squats, I must share an epiphany I had while in Europe using a toilet that had no seat. Ladies, you know where I'm coming from. Wussup with women leaving pee on toilet seats in public restrooms? With the help of a Euro-toilet that offered no place to sit, I finally figured it out: Women are trying to avoid touching the seat for fear of cooties, but their weak quad muscles can't hold them in the squat position long enough; hence the spillage. I feel strangely relieved to have solved this mystery. I used to assume restrooms were haunted by a mournful ghost who flung urine as a symbol of how she was having trouble getting to the Other Side.

Diet mentality holds that weight loss relies on repetition: tuna salad for lunch, 10 minutes on the Exercycle at 15% incline. But it's variety that makes it work, nutritionally and physiologically.

Even if you're exercising regularly, the job isn't done. Every so often (perhaps once a month) you've got to shake things up, not just to stave off mental boredom but to avoid muscle boredom as well. Your muscles get to know the routine and, like that ex-boyfriend of mine who was paralyzed inside a marijuana cloud, start cutting corners in order to get by making as little effort as possible.

You need to shock your body out of its rut by challenging it; that's what cross-training is all about, which in turn accounts for why there are hundreds of specialized sneakers to choose from—one pair for walking, one for racquetball, one for sitting around doing nothing.

If you've been sleepwalking through the same weight-machine circuit over and over and over, it's time to try using free weights while lying on your back across a balance ball (don't strain your neck). Or hey—try some capoeira! Helene will be happy to go with you!

It's exhausting to keep changing up on yourself. Planning fatigue sets in. You'd have to quit your job and spend all your time dreaming up what to do next. Iva did her best to spring new routines on me, the kind where I'd give her the you've-gotta-be-kidding look, eyes narrowed to slits. New routines are hard. They make me crabby.

Riding a white stallion to the rescue was J. Travis, brand manager for NYHRC. I paid full price like any other customer when I joined, but once J. figured out he had a reporter in the house (*"Jami's in the house!"*), one with a weekly weight-loss column, he sprang into action. Soon he was setting me up with photo shoots and new twists on old themes; his crowning achievement was a workout he named Booty Call. One time he marched me down a row of instructors like I was reviewing the troops: Here's Anthony Carillo, he developed Iron Yoga; here's Abigail Sweitzer, she'll show you how to work out with rubber bands (and, for all I know, other office supplies).

I was the only one in Iron Yoga who couldn't stand like a tree. I didn't know which side of the sticky mat goes on the floor. But you've got to try new things even if you look like Bigfoot in the land of the sylphs.

"Next, I'm going to have you kickboxing," announced J., and I wasn't happy to hear it. My Muay Thai teacher was Yuki, an exotic-looking slip of a girl barely old enough to vote. There's nothing private about kickboxing; we did it in a ring in the middle of the gym, which set off panic flashbacks to the tap-dancing class. (*"To the right! I said to the right!"*)

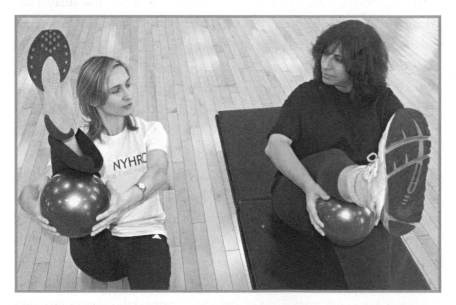

Dina Kozitskaya demonstrates alternate stretches at New York Health & Racquet Club. *(Photo by Tanya Braganti, courtesy New York* Daily News*)*

Yuki wrapped my hands and wrists with athletic tape in a somber ritual that advertised me to the rest of the gym as a pro who was seriously ready to kick ass. Then, embarrassingly, she had to show me over and over how to make a fist properly so I didn't "hit like a girl."

Yuki mostly gets male clients. They like to be seen sparring with her because it's an erotic fantasy—big strong man overpowering delicate Asian flower. But Yuki is no delicate flower. She could have been raised on a military base. *"Is that all you got?"* she screamed when I did a few girlie push-ups and flopped on the mat to rest.

Yes, Yuki, that's all I got. Macho bullying probably gets under the skin of the male clients and whips them into competitive fury—the very sensation they want from a workout, something that strikes a primitive chord from their evolutionary caveman past. (*"You think I no catch bison? Grrr!"*) Me, I looked at Yuki as if she'd asked a rhetorical question. Yes, that's all I got! Can I go home now?

But I learned to kick and punch, and I came out of my first Muay Thai session so elated that I speed-dialed J. and babbled onto his answering machine like I was high on crack. *"I love kickboxing!"* I burbled. "I love the power and the thud, the way it sounds when you connect with the bag at just the right angle! I'm a woman warrior!"

Alas, a woman warrior with a touch of bursitis in her left hip. The kickboxing lessons wound down to a painful end, with an MRI and months of physical therapy in their wake. Plus an all-new humiliation—bursitis turns out to mean inflammation of the fat pads. *Fat pads!*

Okay, what next? Helicopter skiing was out, as was bungee jumping and spelunking. When I say I'm hungry for adventure, I mean *mild* adventure; the Pirates of the Caribbean ride at Disney, preferably with Johnny Depp in my lap.

J. talked me into being Team Leader for an American Cancer Society fundraising run in Central Park; "Join Jami!" blasted the posters he taped to the locker room.

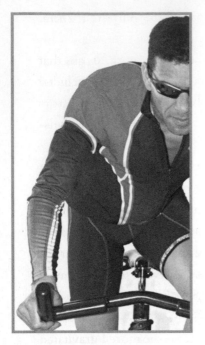

Pablo Toribio, best spin instructor in New York. *(Photo courtesy NYHRC)*

When I was cranky, J. would drag me to something new. It was he who first got me to Pablo Toribio's spin class, especially after I whined how I didn't "get" spin and I didn't know how to stand up on the pedals. Now I take Pablo's class three times a week.

J. almost got me into a kayak for an 18-mile paddle up the Hudson, but (thankfully) it conflicted with my movie-watching schedule.

He also turned me on to Pilates, which I adored for as long as I was willing to pay for sessions on the Reformer machine, something Joseph Pilates invented when he worked up his eponymous method in 1923 to help wounded German soldiers. He built spring-driven machines that are still standard in many Pilates studios, although most of the moves can also be done on floor mats. As a lover of gadgets and technology, I find the equipment intriguing—like the Wundachair, a contraption on which you do spring-loaded handstands (not quite as bad as capoeira but still mighty challenging).

At first glance, the whole Pilates method seemed daft, yet I was strangely hooked. It addresses core strength, flexibility, and alignment, all of which appeal to injured dancers. (The "core," by the way, is the latest hot topic in strength conditioning; they talk about it in hushed tones as if it were something Moses rushed back for: *"Here's the tablets . . . wait, I forgot something!"*)

I told Alycea Ungaro, founder of the RealPilates studio in Tribeca (she also has an outpost at NYHRC) about my bursitis, and we did a rejuvenating workout to strengthen the inflamed area without hurting it. *There, there, my fat pads. Mommy's here.*

Alycea also taught me the "scoop," an important posture for abs that she likened to an ice-cream scoop. Many of her suggestions included food-related visualizations, a welcome relief from those male instructors who equate whatever you do or eat to football fields and manual transmissions. (*"Think of your body as a carburetor!"*)

It's sad that exercise has become—in modern times and as we get older—a chore that needs to be scheduled like a medical checkup. When I was a child, we simply *played*. We raced around, screamed with delight, rode our tricycles, and ran, ran, ran (even though some of us had grandmothers urging us to sit down and conserve our energy for puberty). There was no thought as to how many calories we burned or how much time we logged. Children play. That's what they do.

I wanted to retrieve that sense of play. Like ex-smokers who want to be around other nonsmokers, the more active I became the more I gravitated toward like-minded friends. I met them for walks or workouts instead of brunch. I began to make adult play dates that didn't revolve around meals. I didn't abandon my less aerobic friends, it's just that I wanted more physical activity in my spare time.

Luckily, I have JoAnne—we take long walks through Prospect Park or over the Brooklyn Bridge, although we always fight over whether it's better to eat *before* walking or after. (I'm in the "after" camp; you continue to burn calories long after you've raised your metabolism, and who wants to get moving right after a meal?) My gym buddy Diane Stefani and her husband, Terry, added a bike rack for three on their car to accommodate me; we've taken the bikes out to Bruce's place in the Hamptons and we have dreams of long-weekend bike tours in Vermont.

Helene is always up for anything—biking in Central Park (with one of her toddlers in the kiddie caboose), swimming, capoeira.

Then there's Amanda the Exercise Nazi, in a league by herself. My friendship with Amanda almost ended over a cheeseburger (she wouldn't let me eat it).

When I regained a couple of pounds over one holiday, I knew what to do. It was time for the Exercise Nazi. For a weekend in Connecticut with Amanda, I packed not just a change of socks and T-shirts but enough equipment for sports camp—stuff for running, biking, tennis, ice skating, hiking, and weight training, and, who knows, perhaps a broom for curling. She met me at the train, stopwatch in hand. We sprinted to her car and never stopped moving. We power-walked on the beach. We kayaked. We biked in a sudden downpour. We swam.

That was just the first day.

I was wrung out, faint with exhaustion, broken. All the T-shirts I'd brought were sopping wet. And there was Amanda, still bouncing around looking for a tennis partner and making plaintive "no one will play with me" whines like my cat Buzz.

"I've got *spilkes*," she said, Yiddish for ants in the pants. There's something wrong with that girl.

I was so tired that when Amanda's younger son, Evan, suggested a round of Ping-Pong, I fled in terror. "I've got to renew my car inspection sticker!"

I don't have a car.

But it's amazing how soon complacency sets in. By mealtime at Amanda's, I could have eaten the sofa. True, I had exercised. But my appetite and sense of entitlement remind me of another Sufi tale—again, a long, shaggy-dog story—whose upshot is that a man learns just how overreaching he's been when a wiser man observes, *"Thou hast filled thy belly like a hero."*

And so the delicate dance continues—increase your activity, fill thy belly like a hero, decrease your activity because you're so full you can barely push back from the table, gain back some weight, start over. It's a natural part of the learning process. But it looks as though I'll need to invest in a commuter ticket to Amanda's.

I lost the first 10 pounds through eating smaller portions of better-quality food, making strategic substitutions, and moving around more. I lost the second 10 as I got in touch with some of my warped childhood ideas about food and self-nurture.

During the third set of 10, I began writing the *Daily News* column. Under the pressure of those weekly deadlines and the responsibility to report honestly to my readers, I ramped up the exercise and started researching what made for successful weight loss. Healthy living had truly become a priority, not just something theoretical.

Amanda, who has eaten healthfully most of her adult life (if you discount her insistence that wine is a food group), was delighted I was finally joining her spartan ranks. Obsession loves company. She organized a healthy-retreat weekend along with her childhood chum Blanka at the New Age Health Spa, located near a nature preserve in the Catskills.

On our first morning hike, Amanda sprinted two mountains ahead while I "warmed up." Blanka very sensibly returned to the room, feigning nausea. I stumbled through the underbrush, starting to doubt the wisdom of female bonding; it's so seventies.

While other guests drank herbal tea and did trust-building exercises, each of us pulled out a cell phone and got our exercise by racing around the extensive woodland property trying to get a signal.

I'd been to this same place long ago during my spa-reporting days, back when I was freaking out over hitting 135 pounds. *Can you imagine?* I never thought I'd see the day when I'd be deliriously happy to be down to 200. The place was run back then by a crazy German lady who insisted our bodies could properly be cleansed only through the agency of coffee enemas. They wouldn't let you have caffeine there except up your ass.

Now under different management, the spa is less austere, although I'm still leery of any place that thinks your body is crawling with "toxins" that need to be cleansed or exfoliated or irrigated with colonics, or where the word *juice* is used as a verb ("Yes, I'm *juicing* to get rid of the *toxins*"). But the food was fresh and delicious (they grow their own extensive salad-bar items in a greenhouse), the walks in the woods were inspirational. By Day Two, we were finding that yoga was a nice way to start the day and that Scrabble on the porch at sunset—even without that food group known as wine and even though Blanka has memorized all the two-letter words—is a lovely way to end it. Cell phones forgotten, we were getting to know and appreciate each other in ways we hadn't bothered with before.

"Hey, let's get up at six tomorrow and do an extra hike!" suggested Amanda.

I love Amanda dearly, but I vote her off the island.

40 POUNDS:
UNWISE, BETTER, BEST

There are plenty of things to stare at when you're seated next to Robert Redford at a dinner party. You can stare at his hair, which looks as Sundance Kid as ever, thick with sun-washed highlights. You can stare at his face, still ruggedly handsome despite serving as a walking ad for sunblock and collagen filler.

Me, I chose to stare at his plate. I paid some attention to the man himself, even had a nice chat about the sensuous pleasures of snow. But I was chiefly concerned with what he ate.

Bob—and I think he'd want me to call him Bob—is a compact fellow, and I know from experience that it's instructive to watch how thin people eat. They don't obsess about food (the healthy ones, anyway). They leave a few morsels behind instead of Hoovering it up like the last line of coke of the eighties. Bob can afford to have slave girls drizzle the finest melted chocolate over his naked body, but instead he eats sensibly, remaining movie star slim.

How does he do it?

For one thing, he skis all the time, which burns calories and is easy to schedule when you own so much prime real estate in Utah's Wasatch Mountains. But let's stick to his food choices for now.

★ Readers Weigh In

"I've struggled with weight every day since I can remember and have had some success through that moderation thing, changes in eating habits, etc. But, as with smoking and alcoholism, you're always recovering, never cured."
—E.C., BALI

"My advice? Just beam yourself back into the times of 'Quest for Fire' when fat chicks were de rigueur." —B.R.

"I lost 100 pounds by starting to exercise (walking and bike riding), changing what I ate (I eliminated junk foods and sugary snacks), and learning how to stop when I felt full. It felt great to realize that the clothes I was having trouble fitting into were now falling off me!" —K.T., BROOKLYN

"I started to eat, drink, walk, talk, and think right, and I lost about seven pounds a month. Krispy Kremes are just a glazed glimmer of a memory; like old boyfriends, they did me no good but I can't help thinking about them every so often." —P.S., CINCINNATI

"I've been walking three times a week, and though I haven't seen any significant weight loss, I'm an optimist." —S.K., JAKARTA

"Our weight is a barometer of how we feel about ourselves and how we deal with life. It has to do with what messages we got as youngsters that led us to a system of reward and punishment with food." —N.O., STATEN ISLAND

"I am on a quest to lose about 70 pounds. I was very active up until I reached my 30s and went through a couple of job layoffs and a very destructive relationship. Now I am in Weight Watchers and it works for me." —L.B., ATLANTA

"Cut everything in half!" —C.D.

"Last year, I weighed 307. I'm now down to 244. I'm eating a lot of salads and drinking water like crazy. I freeze a bottle of water every night and take it to work in the morning." —S.R.

"I have struggled with being overweight my whole life. I finally lost 65 pounds in eight months on the Atkins Diet. I have another 25 to go and those are going to be the hardest because I hate to exercise. Who doesn't?" —N.J.

"I was 185 lbs. as a Marine in Vietnam, and found after age 40 I had a real struggle. The mind is still young, but the body starts betraying you by not burning off the same level of food you ate at age 25." —M.S.

"I just hit my 90-pound weight loss mark. When you get hungry during the day: Nuts or trail mix in moderation." —J.B., NEW YORK

I had what he had—the chicken instead of the steak. He left half on his plate; so did I. He picked at his dessert; so did I, even though it was molten chocolate cake. (I excavated the molten part.)

If I eat like Bob, maybe I'll be slim like him. Will I also be a multimillionaire with forever-young hair? I don't think so. For now, I'll settle for imitating healthy eating habits from handy role models, famous or not.

I needed Bob more than ever. I was in what we in the weight-loss trenches call a *high-risk situation*—I was covering the Sundance Film Festival in Utah, a region where they think chicken-fried steak is spa cuisine.

Food is a challenge at film festivals, not just the ones in ski resorts where the phrase "leafy green vegetable" doesn't parse. We won't even go into the bread pudding with vanilla bourbon sauce at the Blind Dog Grill. It's assumed by the restaurants in Park City that the people staying there must be in training for the slalom event and need to coat their arteries with thick gravy and mashed potatoes, just as you'd coat your skin with viscous mud if you were about to swim the English Channel. It's for your own protection.

Dinner options at Sundance usually consist of a side of some wild animal; I think you're encouraged to shoot it yourself and haul the carcass right over to the chef. It's a weird place for a film festival, what with all those sprout eaters alighting from Los Angeles, but the venue was chosen because Redford, who presides, lives close by. Sundance the festival is near Sundance the ski resort because it's convenient for Bob, not because it's the right place to house people for whom "wilderness survival" means burr-grinding your own coffee.

It turned out to be a blessing that the only room I could get on short notice was at a hotel so out of the loop that it was faster and easier to walk two miles to the theaters than to take a succession of three roundabout shuttle buses. Slogging back to the hotel by foot each night on a dark, slushy highway might sound pathetic, but it proved an excellent coping strategy—I actually lost weight during that festival. I like to think my good, close, personal friend Bob would approve.

Each festival offered a new set of high-risk situations: Cannes, with its Champagne parties and indulgent sauces. The Florida Film Festival, where I was a judge for the documentary competition; the motel didn't have a gym and it was too cold at the time to use the outdoor pool, so I roped a fellow juror into driving me over to the YMCA each morning.

At least film festivals offer a semblance of structure. Business trips are easier, foodwise, than vacations.

Take, for example, a ski vacation to Grindelwald, Switzerland, notable for the tonnage of cheese that found its way to my plate. Considering that I was in the land where Heidi gorged on dairy products every time the goats weren't looking, calorie creep was inevitable. I skied the Jungfrau region and swam in the hotel's indoor pool, so I was able to offset at least some of the fondue, Raclette, "cheese toast," and rosti—often described on menus as "low-fat" or "wellfit."

Naysayers

Into any weight-loss paradise a little rain must fall. My newspaper column elicited tons of positive and congratulatory e-mails. And also this:

A woman from Howard Beach wrote to say that, judging by my photo, I must be a "kinky lesbian" and that my weight gain was caused by "too much popcorn while watching dumb femme fatale movies." Despite her belief that I am homosexual, she also assured me I would never get a man because my thighs were too fat.

Another deep thinker and great humanitarian wanted me to know that "most readers are snickering at an overweight film critic" and that "I am not pulling for you to lose weight."

A third reader hoped I'd lose weight "and find employment at a modeling agency" because he didn't care for my movie reviews and would prefer that my energies be redirected.

The Gloomy Guses were few, but when they were mean, they were *mean*. They speculated unkindly about my ethnicity, provenance, politics, and sex life. All reporters get occasional responses of this type when their photos run with their stories, but females tend to get more, and of a more personal nature, and when you're fat, you're really in for it.

Mark Roehling of Western Michigan University found, in a review of twenty-nine research studies, that "overweight persons were subject to discrimination in employment decisions based on body weight." And researchers Puhl and Brownell found "clear and consistent scientific literature showing pervasive bias against overweight people. . . . There is now sufficient evidence of discrimination to suggest it may be powerful and occurs across important areas of living."

But it wasn't easy. Since Grindelwald is located close to Germany, its idea of "health food" is a hearty, starch-thickened stew. No matter what I ordered, the food arrived ensconced in bubbling melted cheese, edges crispy and curled gently to hug the edges of the plate. Melted cheese is a culinary sealant over there, applied with a caulking gun. The aches from a serious day of skiing could only be ameliorated with a deep pot of fondue and a bottomless mug of *gluwein,* a rich, warmed wine with mulled spices and sugar. It was like something out of a Monty Python routine: You were met at the bottom of every ski or toboggan run with an oompah band and a vat containing pig's flesh drowned in cheese.

Plus, mysteriously, a pickle and three cocktail onions.

It was heaven, tastewise. But I gained two pounds on that trip and it took weeks to pry them loose again.

Another vacation that turned me into a health amnesiac was the ski trip to Val di Fassa in the Italian Dolomites. My downfall, as usual, was failure to plan ahead. In the back of my mind—a murky place to be under the best of circumstances—I figured I'd wing it and occasionally partake of the local delicacies. It was, after all, *Italy.* Being so close to Austria (at one time the area was actually part of Austria), Val di Fassa offers some of the same cuisine found in German-inflected Grindelwald—an array of dense, fatty meats, now blanketed not in cheese but in thick cuts of bacon and ham. *Abbondanza!*

Frankly, wrapping a pork chop in bacon is like serving chicken with a soft-boiled egg on the side, a gruesome mother-and-child reunion. Every meat dish, bar none, came corseted in ham, some of it air-dried for resilience and wrapped so snugly and neatly over the main course it was like a plateful of Christmas bundles tied with meaty ribbons and bows.

They had as many specialized names for ham as the Eskimos have for snow. I wish I'd copied them down correctly, but after speck, istrione, and prosciutto, my notes include a ham that roughly translates to "someone

⭐ Hazards of Being a Film Critic

The makers of the *SpongeBob* movie sent me a promotional box of Twinkies. I don't even want to discuss it.

who is passionate about the radio" and another that means "to suffer from." I must go back and improve upon my research.

The mingling of Austrian and Italian cuisine was deadly. My behavior around food while there was—how you say?—*non molto bene*.

Meat platters topped with more meat constituted the main course. But you can't just plunge right in—it could be a shock to the system—so first they soften you up with a huge plate of pasta lacquered with self-stick cream sauce. Bracketing the meal would be an appetizer (perhaps melon and prosciutto to keep the "ham" theme going) and a dessert combining the heaviest elements in the periodic table, like strudel and gelato.

Breakfast and dinner were included in the room rate. (The breakfast buffet offered, oddly, linzer tortes.) So you have to eat them, otherwise . . . I think I hear my grandmother calling from beyond the grave: *"It's money down the drain!"*

That just left lunch.

Skip lunch, you say? Never! My friends Kathie and Hal Aaron had organized the trip, but Hal had then severed

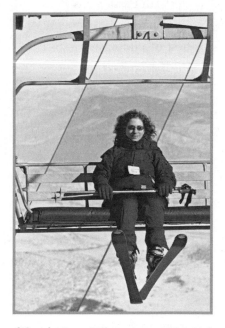

(Photo by Steve Wilson, courtesy New York Daily News)

his Achilles tendon while skiing the week before, and Delta had lost Kathie's luggage and skis. I couldn't very well leave my gracious hosts alone in their pain! So I'd ski half a day, then meet them at La Grotta for pizza and gelato. La Grotta's menu had page upon page describing its pizzas. I had no idea what I was ordering—I'd learned only enough Italian to tell the van driver, "I'd like my beer in a glass"—so I ordered mystery toppings like *bracioletta* or the sublimely named *stinco* (which turned out to be knuckle of veal). *Gorgonzola* needed no translation.

★ Readers: The Moderate

"I have now lost about 140 pounds and I feel wonderful. I did not follow any specific diet, just changed my way of eating. I took it one day at a time, drank lots of water, ate healthy, slowly incorporated exercise back into my life, and everything fell into place from there." —N.J.

Once the groaning pizzas had been packed away with only an occasional crust to betray that food had once occupied the plate, it was time . . . no, not for another ski run, or a trip to town to buy gifts for friends, or a workout at the hotel gym or even a shvitz in the sauna. No, it was time for *gelato,* buckets of it, topped with a sugar-candy mountain of *panna* (cream). In honor of the Austro-Italian connection, I'd ask for my trencher of gelato *"mit schlag,"* the Austrian way of saying "please clog my arteries with *panna.*"

Hal is an excellent cook, and he and Kathie appreciate the eros of fine dining. There may be people in the world who eat simply because they must, but dining with Hal and Kathie is like worshipping at the altar of divine edibles. They don't go for just anything, mind you, only *great* food—the right yeasty pizza dough, *stracciatella* gelato whose delicate whorls of chocolate shavings startle from within a swirling tunnel of vanilla.

The gelato, by the way, was served in a flared Murano glass bowl, as befits such treasure.

The third time we met at La Grotta for lunch, K&H's friend Tony came along. Tony, like Hal, is a black-diamond skier who burns calories like rocket fuel on the slopes, but I've rarely witnessed the pleasured abandon with which he orders and consumes. He drenched his pizza with olive oil, then pinched up a slice with his hand, American-style, and salted it as if about to bake it in one of those rock-hard salt crusts that you have to hammer open. We'd barely finished our pizzas, with their kaleidoscope of fleshy, marbled toppings, when Tony magisterially ordered *"stracciatella grande."* We all followed suit, only to find that special dessert pails had to be located just to accommodate this treat, like finding a sling to hoist those super-heavy people from their beds when they need hospitalization. Our mountainous desserts were so high they had their own weather system, and their distant peaks were capped *mit schlag.*

Down below, among gelati boulders whose size suggested the carvings of Easter Island, the weather was clear and cold. Up top it was cloudy *mit schlag,* with low visibility and, if eaten in its entirety, a high mortality rate.

I ate it in its entirety. Then I took a nice long Italian nap, the kind that takes you right through to dinner.

Anytime you leave home and the safety of your routine, food becomes problematic: midnight buffets on cruises, second helpings thrust upon you by well-meaning hosts. Living in a plastic bubble begins to sound mighty attractive.

Eventually, I learned how to handle high-risk situations from the folks at the Hilton Head Health Institute, a spa in South Carolina with a medically sound program and an effective way of teaching it.

I haven't always liked spa vacations. There was a short period in my early newspaper career where I covered them for the travel section. Still in my twenties, I was thin and didn't need a spa. Nor did I see the point of those pampering-type facilities where the guests are matrons whose husbands don't touch them enough; hence the popularity of booking massages every day.

★ Readers: Protein Girl

"I'm like Henry VIII with protein, just short of waving a turkey leg in the air. I'll get a triple-decker corned beef-turkey-coleslaw sandwich at the deli but have them hold the bread. It's fascinating how cooperative and creative restaurants will be when you tell them you can't eat bread." —NAME WITHHELD ON REQUEST

I didn't even *like* massages. I had to learn to appreciate them. To me, "massage" meant exotic-oil foreplay with a boyfriend, not the chain-smoking old lady with the spider-veined hands who took a look at me on the massage table of one big-deal Florida spa and croaked, "How long ago was the surgery, dearie?"

Ah, yes. The surgery. Again the luck of the genetic draw: I have great skin and a superb blood-lipid profile, but I also had my gallbladder out at age twenty-eight, same as my mom, even though I was slender at the time. (Gallbladder disease is usually associated with being overweight.)

Considering my age, I've had more than my share of trips to the hospital. Each time they take something out, I make the same nervous joke about how this will reflect nicely on the scale. Do wisdom teeth count? The Elective Surgery Diet isn't as funny as I'd like to think, because I'll bet there are women who would go for it.

At spa after spa, I suffered silently through torturous massages. I didn't get what the fuss was about—until years later, at Utah's Red Mountain spa, which started out under its original, vegan owner as a bare-bones military-style encampment. If you wanted a snack at night, your only option was a cold boiled potato in order to teach you the difference between physical hunger (during which you'll eat the potato) and mouth hunger, or desire (never mind, you were rather hoping for a cream puff). The spa's focus, then as now, is on sunrise hikes in the gorgeous, rust-colored canyons. But as the owners changed, they've gradually upgraded from boot camp to something more pampering (they no longer force you out of your room at 6:30 A.M.), and I suddenly realized during a treatment for sore muscles that the masseur was doing tricky, flirtatious little moves with his knuckles that he must have spent weeks dreaming up. It was endearing how he was trying so hard to arouse me. He whispered hoarsely when he asked me to turn over, grabbed a hank of my hair and pulled it gently but firmly in a cross between scalp massage and Neanderthalism.

Now I get it. I giggled and immediately booked massages for every night of my stay.

When the publicist for the Hilton Head Health Institute (HHHI) called and asked if I wanted to check out the place, I thought it would be another one of those pay-someone-to-stroke-you spas, and I wasn't altogether against it. But much more gratifyingly, HHHI is a serious place that offers a science-based program for losing large amounts of weight. No fads or gimmicks, just the facts, ma'am. It's like going to weight-loss school (you even get a mock diploma). It's not a one-off experience that fades the moment you get within nostril-distance of Cinnabon (700 calories for a small Cinnabon pastry, by the way).

The current owner is John Schmitz, a self-made man who experienced a wakeup call of his own when blood started running from his nose one day. It spurred him to bail out of the corporate world—is any job worth having if it makes blood run from your nose? He bought the spa and changed his life. His new philosophy? *If it's shiny, don't eat it.*

Schmitz likes to describe how he moved from I'm Deprived and Pissed Off all the way to Righteous Superiority. Once he started losing weight, he wasn't content to eat his grilled fish and steamed broccoli without commenting on everyone else's food. "You're not going to eat *that!*" he'd cry in dismay, calling cheese "tar for the veins" and hurling unpleasantries. "I was totally obnoxious," he now admits.

⭐ Readers: The Resolute

"I decided I would lose 150 pounds. I was a fat baby, grew into a fat child, became a fat adult. But I made up my mind not to treat this as a diet but as a life makeover. I've since lost 15 pounds. I've decided to use the same tenacity that got me through other endeavors in life." —S.S.

He got over it. When I visited him in Arizona, he fried up bacon for breakfast. John is willing to exercise five hours a day (not an exaggeration) to keep his weight down during the times he eats like that; for all I know, he was just showing off for visitors. An aerialist does a loop-de-loop and a spa owner shows he can eat bacon for breakfast and still maintain his weight.

After a rasher of crispy bacon, he marched me eight miles up the steep incline of a nearby canyon, certainly a more pleasant exercise experience than running on a poorly maintained treadmill whose readout keeps blinking: *Lubricate belt*. But I, for one, could never keep up that level of exercise. The day would come—probably Tuesday—when my weight would creep up like a coyote on an unsuspecting hiker in the Arizona canyons.

The best advice for daily weight regulation I ever got was from HHHI, and bacon had nothing to do with it. Chief among the instructors there is Bob Wright, director of Lifestyle Education, who looks to me more like a

Midwestern football jock than a guy with a master's in health ed who does the grocery shopping for his family. ("Honey, have you read the nutritional label on this can of garbanzo beans? It'll blow your mind!") Bob has a steel-trap memory for peer-reviewed studies of how many biceps curls a ninety-year-old must do to prolong his life by 10 minutes. And he makes it all fascinating, even the part about trans-fats.

In a series of lectures—HHHI packs the schedule with an alternating current of exercise and informational classes—Bob put into medical context all the things I'd intuited about healthy living and weight loss: habit changing, meal planning, metabolism goosing, healthy snacking, reasonable goals.

During the wrap-up session, Bob reiterated his trademark coping phrase for high-risk situations: *Unwise, better, best*. I'll say this for Bob: For all his wonderful qualities, he's not much of a sloganeer. It's unclear how many of the catchphrases used at HHHI are Bob's invention or holdovers from the original program by founder Peter Miller. Some might even be cobbled from the nutritional stylings of Dr. Phil, who advises in *Dr. Phil McGraw's Ultimate Weight Solution* to "stop living like a lazy slug." When the Department of Health and Human Services says Calories Count, it's simple and elegant and has the whiff of a pun—even if they came to this sensible conclusion late in the game yet act as if they've discovered the ancient civilization of Atlantis. Meanwhile, Bob continues to come up with phrases that don't exactly trip off the tongue, like "If you fail to plan, you're planning not to succeed."

Nevertheless, "unwise, better, best" is a winner. In dangerous eating climes—when traveling or under stress, for example—the goal is not to be perfect but to make choices along a spectrum of unwise, better, best. At the Cannes Film Festival, "better" meant one mini-éclair at the buffet, whereas "unwise" would have been a plateful. (The fact that Will Smith and the alarmingly skinny Angelina Jolie were one table over helped my resolve; I didn't want Will saying, "You know, Angie, the Mediterranean is lovely this time of year, but what's with that chick and the éclairs?")

There's no judgment attached to unwise, better, best. It's about making a reasonable effort under difficult circumstances. Or as my reader Robin put it, "Always remember that having four Milky Ways is better than the six or eight you had before."

This ties into another HHHI precept, "degrees of on," in which you are never "on" program or "off" program, merely attached to a different extent at all times. Ideally, you strive for the upper end, where "on" is a neon halo. But as long as you're on to some degree, there's a spread of what's acceptable in terms of calories, behavior, and exercise adherence. Being connected to a healthy lifestyle to some degree at all times is more efficient in the long run than being "perfect" a fraction of the time. The problem with rigidity (aside from alienating friends) is that when you fail to meet lofty, arbitrary, self-imposed standards, the tendency is to give up entirely and go back to bed with the cellophane wrappers from Hostess cupcakes crinkling beneath you.

You can calculate "degrees of on" from many angles and fine-tune accordingly. Calorie-wise, you can figure a high end of how much you can eat while maintaining your weight—somewhere around 1800 or 2000 calories a day for me. The low end should be no less than 1200 calories, below which you'll barely have the strength to chew a stick of sugar-free gum.

★ Readers: The Risk Taker

"I lost 67 pounds and reached my ideal weight. I probably did it all wrong. However, I made modifications which I still use. Instead of eating a couple of slices of cheesecake at the end of the day, I opt for three or four Edy's fruit bars at a reasonable 80 calories a pop. Maybe I am in the danger zone here, but so far it's working. Also, there is no such thing as too much exercise!" —E.G., BROOKLYN

The low end shouldn't be any—or at least not much—lower than your resting metabolism, the amount of energy that your body normally needs simply to exist. I had my resting metabolic rate tested at HHHI with a device called the BodyGem. You breathe into it for 15 minutes and it reports exactly how many calories you use per day if you don't do anything special, such as taking the stairs two at a time (like *that* would happen). The readout tells you how much energy your body needs just to maintain itself; above that, fluctuations in weight depend on how much food you take in over your requirement, factored against how much exercise you do to burn it off.

You can also figure your resting metabolic rate mathematically, which in my case yielded almost precisely the same results as with the BodyGem.

I assumed that by being fat I had an advantage—I probably burned thousands of calories just going for the mail. But I was wrong. At 200 pounds, accounting for moderate exercise up to five times a week, my resting metabolic rate was 1420 calories. That meant I had to eat between 1200 and 1600 calories a day (along with a supplement of exercise) to see slow, steady weight loss. That's not much food—a meal at a generic diner can easily run you 1600 calories unless you fill it with soups and vegetables, which are full of water and take up a lot of volume. (That's the basic theory behind Volumetrics, that you can eat more when you choose lower-calorie items that are bulky and filling.)

Your resting metabolism can seem pitifully low, meaning that even when you eat like a bird it's possible to gain weight. You can raise that rate by building muscle through exercise, but your resting metabolic rate is never going to be a tremendous number. There's a small window between how many calories you need and how many are too many. The goal is to "eat sensibly," but you still have to stay cognizant of how many calories you draw from the daily bank.

Behaviorally, here's what you do: Define your goals and map a course for achieving them. As Bob takes pains to point out, these aren't weight goals, like "I want to lose 15 pounds in three days, and my strategy is to sit in a sauna until I'm carried off to the ER." My goal at Cannes included the specific hope of making it past the patisserie located next to my hotel. In past years, I'd stop in as routinely as I did at the hotel lobby to check for messages, and when things got rough—deadlines, boring movies, foot-in-mouth disease at a cocktail party—I'd squirrel away éclairs in my room. Even when things went well, I felt like I was in the trenches; *"Incoming!"* someone would yell before lobbing a fusillade of pastries.

Another specific new goal at Cannes was to go to the gym—again, just to keep a sense of connection to my usual routine so it wouldn't pull apart later like the pastry layers of a *millefeuille*. My hotel, the evocatively named Modern Waikiki, was lucky to have a one-person elevator, let alone a fitness center. To find a gym, I had to go across the street to the Majestic Hotel, which charged a majestic day rate of 25 euros. I went every other day for complete cardio and weight workouts, often alongside the Russian director Nikita Mikhalkov (*Burnt by the Sun*), whose work I admire even though he yelled at me in bad French to close the windows of the gym. What, no fresh Mediterranean air? Wasn't he accustomed to the frozen tundra or the steppes of his homeland?

⭐ Readers: The Actress

Kim Sandstrom of Oregon is boxing, rafting, and shooting hoops, a far cry from when she was 80 pounds heavier and bedridden with medical problems.

"I used walkers and canes to get around. . . . I began a new way of living and thinking, eventually eliminating sugar and white flour and eating more lean proteins, vegetables and better-quality grains and fats," wrote

Sandstrom, who, with her husband, Commander John Sandstrom, founded the Hillsboro Actors Repertory Theatre.

After going from a size 2X to a size 4–6, "I am now living the life I love in theater, performing, directing, writing, etc. I am now 134 pounds and within four pounds of a goal that was heretofore considered unreachable and unrealistic. I feel great and I feel powerful . . . yep, I do!"

Colleagues pitched in with suggestions for where to score quick salads. Indie film reporter Mary Glucksman was really helpful until she told me where to find free dark-chocolate squares. *This is not the kind of advice the Incredible Shrinking Critic needs.* And anyway, Mary, they weren't on the fourth floor of the Palais like you said.

At restaurants, I ordered grilled sea bream (a local fish) instead of steak frites, salade Niçoise instead of Caesar. And French yogurt is to die for.

I needed to report in for my weight-loss column. Fortunately, every pharmacy in France has a scale. When you insert a half-euro coin, it spits out a receipt that gives your weight in kilograms, your height in centimeters, and the number of calories you really ought to be eating. I expected a hand (with a French manicure) to reach out from the machine and slap my face: *Stop eating ʒee food!*

Pascal at my hotel did the math for me, changing kilograms to pounds. After two weeks in the South of France, faced with every temptation from the overeater's torture pantry, I hadn't gained an ounce.

With Cannes as a point of comparison, I can now look back at a high-risk situation like the trip to Val di Fassa and analyze what I could have done better. One of the cornerstones of weight loss is learning from mistakes. If we were to examine my slide down the ski slope of gluttony like lab technicians examining a beaker for sediment, we'd find that the simple problem during the Italy trip was lack of planning.

I'd gotten smug. I'd made the mistake of thinking like a novice stock investor that past performance guarantees future earnings. I'd started to think that I could eat anything I wanted and easily snap back to healthy habits. So I'll just suck it up and admit that while in Val di Fassa I forgot all about unwise, better, best. As Bob Wright would say, "If you fail to plan, you're planning not to succeed."

For Cannes, I planned ahead with military precision and the help of my food wranglers—e-mail support from Bob, consultations with the Nutrition Twins, extra workouts with Iva. We strategized about how to protect my flank from flank steaks and my rear from snack attacks. I used "unwise, better, best" to gauge my behavior. I stayed conscious of "degrees of on" to maintain a behavioral connection to my regular routine.

Learning from mistakes is not only about putting on the hair shirt. Val di Fassa was not an utter disaster, despite those lunches. I may have eaten as if I'd come from a POW camp where all they gave you was bugs and dirt, but there was still the matter of "degrees of on." During the Italy trip, there was just enough "on"—the pulse was weak, but detectable—because whilst filling my belly like a hero, I was also skiing.

Every day. Hours at a time.

It was in Italy that I finally graduated to the intermediate *piste*. I was so sick with fear I wanted to throw up or cry, even as schools of four-year-olds streamed past me with their brightly bobbed ski hats prancing in the sunlight. Hmmph, must be their low center of gravity.

Crying and vomiting would have been a lovely way to impress my ski instructor, Milka, who spoke no English but liked to gesture to the intermediate trails, look at me meaningfully, and giggle.

I also went to the hotel gym. The Italian who presided over it watched me, frowning. He didn't speak any *l'Inglese,* and at every exercise I tried,

⭐ Readers: The Better Half

"I lost 18.6 pounds in eight weeks on Weight Watchers. I am trying to lose weight not only for myself but also for my three kids. My husband—ah, let's forget about him. He thinks he's svelte at 5-10 and 240 pounds." —J.

he shook his head disapprovingly. My lateral raises were all wrong. My triceps kickbacks were a thing of disgust. My sweat was so copious he furiously mopped the equipment I'd touched, using my own towel so as not to sully the clean ones reserved for less sweaty guests. No matter how much weight I lifted or how raised my pulse, I couldn't impress this guy.

Maybe he didn't like fat girls, even ones who had lost 40 pounds.

You can't exercise off every calorie once you decide to strap yourself in for the *stracciatella grande*. But you can mitigate the damage. I gained only two pounds during that two-week pig-out in Italy. The real triumph was that I used "degrees of on" even when everything seemed hopeless. "Being on or off isn't a calorie thing, it's a behavioral thing," Bob explains. "It's a feeling of connection rather than a calorie issue. It's about a sense of having managed the situation. If you give yourself an expectation under those very high-risk situations that cannot be met, when it's not met, you're back to 'forget it.'"

I use the techniques I learned at HHHI every day. The first "real-world" test came the day I left the spa, all fired up to be the healthiest-living person on the planet. I stepped into the Savannah airport for my flight home and was confronted with a sight more frightening than the empty ship gliding into port in the vampire classic *Nosferatu*—a food court, with nary a healthy snack in sight. Burger King, Pizza Hut, all the usual suspects were represented. Finally, at a kiosk that had the word *healthy* in its name (even though that turned out to be a misnomer), I chose a turkey and cheese sandwich from which I extracted and rejected the mayo-spackled cheese. I'm not fond of mayo, and cheese, you know, is a condiment.

As Bob might put it in his inimitable way, it wasn't the best, but it was better than unwise.

50 POUNDS:
SEXUAL HEALING

I had the wrong idea about love, perhaps from the beginning.

> *Diary entry, age 7:* I am at home and writing with rose flower pens. I had a bacon sandwich for supper, and for dessert had chocolate milk with Nestle's Quik and pound cake. First I drank coffee, then Bosco, and now Nestle's Quik. I keep on thinking from "Tarzan and the She-Devil" that Jane is saying, "Tarzan! TARZAN!"

This was followed two weeks later by an entry regarding a made-for-TV Disney movie called *The Scarecrow of Romney Marsh*, with Patrick McGoohan dressed in burlap Zorro mask as he valiantly rode to the rescue of poor folk being conscripted into the king's navy. It was a two-

Wednesday, January 29, 1964

29th day — 337 days follow

Dear Anne, I am at home and writing with hose Flower pens. I had a baken sawndwich for supper, and for dessert I had chaclet milk with Nestlys Quik and pound cake. First I drank coffie, then Boscoo and now Nestlys Quik. I alsq did my homework. I did it 3 after 7 exactly. I keep on thinking from Tarzan and the she ere that Jane is saying Tarzan TARZAN. love,

parter of he-man derring-do that stirred hormones I didn't know a seven-year-old could have. After the first installment aired, my diary read:

Today I watched Mr. Ed, Lassie, and Walt Disney. Walt Disney was the best. It was "Scarecrow." But it didn't scare crows, it scared people!

Fair enough. The future film critic honing her craft.

By the following week, the movie had begun to sink in:

> "Scarecrow" is finished from Walt Disney. I'm crying over that. I want him back. Scarecrow, Scarecrow, Scarecrow, Scarecrow, the men all feared his name, but the country folk loved him just the same. Scarecrow, Scarecrow!

Scarecrow. *Uh-oh.*

I don't read romance novels. I don't attend Renaissance Fairs or light fragrant candles to entice gentleman callers. I don't try to make myself girlish or mysterious. I only learned to apply makeup, begrudgingly, in my early thirties, because the occasional formal event is unavoidable. Still, my view of what constitutes "romantic" was encrusted in the childhood ovens of hyperventilating melodramas about manly heroes and silent suffering and women who faint prettily into well-muscled arms.

What is love? It's *Wuthering Heights,* where the only man who loves you like you should be loved can only express it after you're dead. It's *Gone With the Wind,* where drunken Rhett promises to kiss you like you should be kissed—"and often!"—and then proves it by hauling you to the boudoir against your will. It's swashbuckler Errol Flynn, square-jawed Burt Lancaster, anything with Alfred Drake on Broadway, brawny chests. As Dorothy Dandridge sang in *Carmen Jones,* "Dat's love!"

> *January 11, 1966:* We played Sexy Barbie. Woo-woo! P.S.: My favorite subject is horses. My favorite books are Black Stallion books by Walter Farley. P.P.S.: I'm listening to Carmen Jones. It's great!

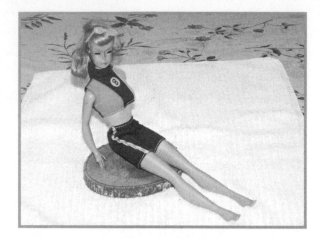

March 2, 1966: Dear BLACK STALLION, Bonfire, Black Minx, Sultan, I have read most of your books. I love you. I wish I owned a horse. I love horses. I give you permission to look in the rest of my Diary to see my drawings of you. I wish I could see a movie called "The Black Stallion."

I got my wish for *The Black Stallion* in 1979, courtesy of director Carroll Ballard. Meanwhile, love—when it wasn't between girl and horse—was mostly what I learned at the movies, because I sure wasn't getting instruction at home. Today, in my capacity as a movie critic, I think it's preposterous that there are people who mistake what's onscreen for real life. Yet that's often how I felt growing up. When I was too young to know better, I asked my mother whether Patty Duke had to stay up late to film *The Miracle Worker;* I thought she was really inside the TV box, waiting patiently in real time for the commercials to stop interrupting.

And so I hoped that Tarzan would one day hop a vine for me. I had the

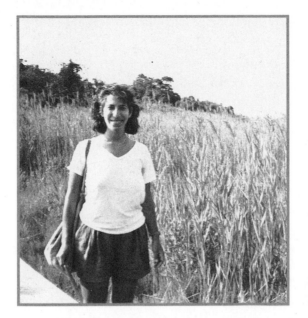

Age 29: 125 pounds, but the clock is ticking.
(*Photo by Amanda Low*)

wrong idea, and I didn't challenge it until . . . um . . . let's just say I'm looking into it.

My romantic relationships, by and large, have sucked. There were exceptions, of course—like Mark, a gentle sweetheart with whom I've remained friends. Not all of my exes are bad people, even though they weren't right for me, and even though a couple of them are Lying, Cheating Scum (LCS, in case I have need of mentioning them again).

Mostly I chose badly, gravitating toward the bad boys. The ones who loved women were great in the sack, but . . . they loved women! *Other* women! The guys who were brooding and remote had all of Heathcliff's worst qualities. (Did Heathcliff have any good ones, aside from looking like the young Laurence Olivier?)

To be fair, I was no picnic either. I could be moody, self-absorbed, oppositional. I was emotionally immature, hiding it as best I could behind intellectual acuity.

In any case, the nice, decent guys never got to me fast enough, pushed aside by the stronger sperm swimming upstream, the ones who wanted to peer down my shirt with a Hubble telescope. I didn't choose wisely despite ample warning signs.

"What's *that?*" one boyfriend asked with disgust, pointing to a freckle defacing my arm. The guy had acne bigger than his dick, and he's worried about a freckle?

My friend Larry had dating advice that I steadfastly ignored. "You'll never be happy until the day you face who you really are," he'd say.

"Which is?"

"A nice girl from Queens."

Ecchhh, as *Mad* magazine would say. The thought was appalling. I wanted to be dangerous! A vixen! Ann-Margret! Someone not to be trifled with! I wanted to be a Jet or a Shark, leaping gymnastically across the playground with switchblade between my teeth!

That probably explains my attraction to Ralph McRotten. There's no discussion of excessive weight gain without examining the contributing factors, and Ralph McRotten made a very generous contribution.

Was it love? Dependency? The handcuffs? What was it all about, Ralphie?

That relationship, in my mid twenties, marked a transition in how I chose to process raw emotion. Before that, when a man did me wrong, I did what any normal girl would do—starved myself or came down with a wilting case of mononucleosis. The McRotten experience introduced me to an exciting new option: When the party's over, that's when the real chowdown begins.

Don't worry. As I discuss my ex-boyfriends, I'll try to take the high road. (Note to self: Go on MapQuest. Locate high road.)

I'd love to sit McRotten down and get his take on the whole fiasco. But he seems to regard me even today as a crazy lady—me, who only bitch-slapped him once! (And that was because he failed to mention he was secretly married and had a baby.) When I passed him on the street a few years ago, he pretended to sneeze so he could turn away and hide his face. I wouldn't have even noticed him except the sneeze was so exaggerated, like a street mime whose silence is a scream for attention. Even when I realized it was him, I didn't break stride; a man who'd rather feign a sneeze than say hello probably isn't going to have much to say.

During our yearlong, star-crossed relationship, Ralph was heavy into two things—me and drugs. Not necessarily in that order. I wasn't opposed to a nice Quaalude or two back in the day, but Ralphie was in a different drug class entirely; on one vacation, he packed his "works"—for shooting up—as proudly as I'd packed silk tap pants from Victoria's Secret.

I can relate to the rush that drugs provide because Ralph was my drug. I was twenty-four and he was seven years older, just older enough that his experience and worldliness seemed fascinating and inexhaustible to me. He'd point at an atlas and say he'd lived in a small village here, a small village there . . . who knows when or why? Or even if? How many small villages could he have lived in? I hung on his every anecdote, even the boring one about the time he borrowed a book from a transsexual. The dynamics of our relationship cannily turned on a Morse Code of give and take—he'd shower me with I-love-you's, then stand me up. It created a Pavlovian expectation; since every pain was followed by a soothing kiss, it got so I'd look forward to the pain, and in fact mistook the pain for love, an emotional substitution that was not wholly unfamiliar to me from various childhood incidents.

I knew—in that shadowy, not fully articulated way that women know—that my boyfriend was cheating and lying. (LCS alert!) But I was so naïve about relationships (*Heathcliff! Rhett!*) that I didn't believe I

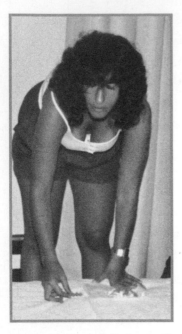

The "cunning outfit," size Small, starting to get tight one year and 7 pounds later. *(Photo by Susan Pivnick)*

was allowed to ask for more, or say no, or get up and leave. Imagine the raccoon that needs to be told by his fellow raccoons how to wash shiny objects in the river! No one ever showed me how to wash the shiny objects—all my friends were in semiabusive relationships of their own at that age—so I stayed with Ralph, clinging, tumbling into an abyss of need.

At first, I was my best self when I was with him. In the safety of his reiterated love and adoration, I was funny, smart, sexy, confident. I loved me when I was with him.

Later, I was my worst self, fulminating with rage. I hated me without Ralph. When Ralph left, he seemed to take away my access to the self I recognized.

Ralph claimed to dabble in the Dark Arts, an assertion to which I nodded with slack-jawed belief as I did to all his boasts about his nature and abilities. He pronounced me an incubus. I had to look it up. What he meant was succubus, an evil female spirit that sucks the life out of men by screwing them in their sleep. Nice.

Anyway, what kind of self-respecting dabbler in the Dark Arts doesn't know his succubus from his incubus?

I remember what I wore pre-, during, and post-Ralph. Everything was size Small. The night he stood me up at the roof party on Front Street, I wore the most adorable French Connection navy short-shorts with a white, clingy, spaghetti-strap Betsey Johnson top, sans bra. My friends regarded me with a combination of sympathy and disgust as my eyes wheeled in every direction to seek out Ralph, for surely he would come.

He didn't. I lay in bed that night still dressed in my cunning little out-fit as if laid out in wedding regalia, a bride abandoned, perhaps dead.

When you feel cherished and understood, it's like speeding down an open road, wind in hair, endless possibilities on the horizon. When all that is taken away, it's like riding with Billy Joel behind the wheel. *Watch out for the tree!* I'm not sure if what I felt for Ralph could technically be called love. But when I was with him, I sure as hell loved *me*, the self that I could only access through the agency of Ralph's high-beam love lights. Maybe *I* was my drug of choice, not Ralph.

The last time I saw Ralph during our dating days, he was fleeing in the night. Since we were on an island at the time and the ferries had stopped running, it was spooky. Did he sleep in the dunes? Did he swim to the mainland, buoyed by coke and paranoia? I wore Ralph's mannish under-wear to bed in a fetishistic attempt to reclaim him, while keeping a kitchen knife under the pillow just in case he crept back in the night to murder me.

Ah, the days of wine and roses!

We'd been sharing a cabin with JoAnne, who had just ended a long-term relationship of her own, plus JoAnne's perpetually vague mother ("Where did that nice Ralphie go?"), and the morose Bill, whose girl-friend Vicky had just dumped him. Bill would stare vacantly at the van-ishing point between sea and sky, his hand trailing on the beach, and intone, *"Vicky liked sand."* Everyone in that house was miserable or con-fused or hiding a kitchen knife under the pillow.

My wise friend Larry repeated patiently and often that in relationships, love is necessary but not sufficient. But all I could think of were Ralph's whispered endearments and brimming eyes; *this* was love! *Heathcliff* love!

Après Ralphie, *le déluge.* I'm not saying he forced me to eat, because there's no one-to-one correlation between people who piss you off and the weight you subsequently gain to get back at them. (And that works *so* well.) But there was no place for my grief to go. I was already doing the usual things—acting out, being a pain in the ass, going over every microscopic detail of the relationship as I searched for signs and portents. What else could I do?

I ate.

The groundwork had been laid—ignorance of nutrition, lack of a regimen, not knowing or caring how to cook, a tendency toward melancholy and drama, and the supersonic snacking techniques learned during all-nighters at college, when excess in all things (drinking, eating, studying, sex) was applauded. On the exercise side, disco was dying and those group outings to after-hours dance palaces dried up. Now, marinated in Ralphie misery, I had no bursts of heart-pumping activity to take my mind off the breakup or at least burn a few calories. There was only food. The solace of chewing.

About seventeen years after Ralph fled into the dunes, a year after his fake sneeze on a Manhattan street, I bumped into him again. When you imbue someone with that much power over you, it's alarming and also a relief to see that the formerly beloved suffers from ordinariness. His face seemed fallen, his nostrils pinched and collapsed from that old coke habit. It was clear—oh, so clear!—that he still thought of me as unstable, and I resent it. But what can I do? The more you insist that you're normal, the crazier you sound. He talks to me in measured tones as if he's got one finger on the panic button.

We had some polite chitchat—how are you, how has your life been? He'd given up drinking and drugging. I'd given up magical thinking; I no longer believed his stories about evil spirits wafting after him. I was neither succubus nor incubus, and Ralph held no power over me now.

But I did feel one powerful emotion—shame. Those sexy little shorts and stretchy little top were about 100 pounds ago. I looked on Ralph's ruined, melted face, wondering how in the world I could have thought he was the be-all and end-all, and he probably thought the same thing looking back at me.

★

I'm surprised I didn't get fat earlier. My heart broke with such regularity it was like the uncle with the trick elbow who can pop it out of joint to amuse party guests.

If yo-yo dieting messes up the metabolism (it doesn't, but I still like to think so), then frequent start-stop relationships ruined my ability to choose men wisely and conduct myself properly. I was hooked on wild, furious breakups and whatever chemical or enzyme they pumped into the bloodstream. I was like people who mutilate themselves—the jolt of breaking up with someone made me feel alive.

Miserable, but alive.

Sometimes they broke up with me, sometimes I broke up with them. Whoever was more needy inevitably got the boot. Whenever a boyfriend showed excessive emotional need, I became—as Thomas Hobbes said in a different context—nasty, brutish, and short. Having been through the Ralph wringer, you'd think I'd cut the poor boys some slack. But I was contemptuous of boyfriends who submitted their jugulars as a sign of appeasement. There's a manipulative aspect to it; "sensitive" is nice, but when someone breaks into tears at the uncanny moment when you're about to get to the heart of some difficult relationship issue, it's crafty indeed, because you can't very well crush a tearful person beneath your heel and walk away.

When it came to love, half the time I'd be—as the *New York Times* would put it in their fundraising drive—one of the Neediest Cases. The other 50 percent of the time, it was the guy who was the craven one while I took on the role of torturer. Let's see if I've got this straight: When a boyfriend is too needy, I dump him. When *I'm* too needy, it's a noble sign of romantic yearning, something that imbues me with color and stature.

I was under the impression that making scenes in public was the ideal expression of my passion for life and my tender vulnerability. There was

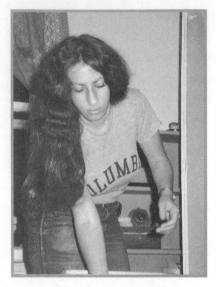

(Photo by Susan Pivnick)

hardly a place on the Columbia University campus where I hadn't made a scene over some college sweetheart—a breakup near the Sundial, a tearful reunion on the Low Library steps, a dramatic renunciation on Furnald Lawn.

Only now, looking back, do I wince. I may have genuinely felt a sense of abandonment during and after those breakups, but was it really about these particular men? Did I have any real feeling for them aside from rage at having been deserted, traded in for someone I assumed was prettier, smarter, more agile in bed? (Code words for thinner?)

It doesn't take a Ph.D. in psych to see the pattern behind my disdainful treatment of men who worshipped me: We hate in others what we hate in ourselves. When it came to love—or "love"—my behavior was its own little engine, fed by fantasy and insecurity. No one had prepared me for interpersonal relationships, only for the schoolwork and tests at which I excelled. My bailiwick was the nonhuman; perhaps it still is. Computers and books, yes; playing well with others, no.

So I was mean to the guys who adored me, inconsolable when dumped. I felt powerless. Anorexia has a lot to do with women trying to control *something* in their lives, when their bodies are the only clay they can get their hands on. Overeating was also a twisted attempt at control, but without the purge, where was the payoff?

Despite a trail of failed relationships and an onslaught of poundage, I didn't stop dating. But by the time 210 pounds rolled around, I can't say I was really into it. It was a relief not to have a relationship to tend or all the triage that comes with the inevitable breakup. It was a relief not to get naked. I still had occasional lovers, including a longtime, on-and-off one who offered to have sex with me for every pound I lost. We did that for about five pounds, and it was amusing—in fact, it was rather hot, especially the time I was draped upside down over the back of a (sturdy) sofa—but it became something of a chore. If I lost a pound, gained it back, and lost it again, did that mean we should have sex twice? The bookkeeping was confusing. Sex-for-pounds sounds intriguing, but in reality you can't put strings on sex or it's not sexy.

As I lost weight, though, I got to a point where I was anxious to road-test the equipment. Just after the 50-pound mark, I suddenly found myself in a relationship. I must have made peace with something inside, because I no longer felt that dating was fraught with problems. It seemed . . . appealing. I found I was no longer interested in bad boys and head cases, addicts and gamblers. The least hint of mental problems or spinelessness turned me off completely. By examining what was right and wrong with me, I'd also, unconsciously, been examining what was worthwhile in others. For the first time I could honestly say I wanted what Salt-N-Pepa rapped about, a mighty good man.

That first man was good in a number of ways, but the Crazy Radar started blipping early on. He was a little *too* into me. It was claustrophobic. On the second date, he tearfully professed his love. On the third date, he said he knew we'd get married. By the fifth date, he was acting weird and suspicious, checking up on me, telephoning at inappropriate hours, and asking strange questions. And drinking too much.

I think being a movie critic is hazardous to my social life. Movies promote this kind of behavior as appropriate, a consummation devoutly to be wished. In real life, it's the behavior of a stalker.

Which he was. I called a lawyer.

It's too bad, because the sex was damn good, proving once again that life is so, so unfair.

Almost by definition, though, you can't have good sex in a bad relationship. At least the interlude was a nice reminder that being fat doesn't mean getting cheated in the sack. And I can tell you, sex is every bit as good fat as thin. I've had it both ways, as they say, and I'm giving it to you straight. I just hope I don't have to date psychopaths to get this much stimulation in the future.

There's no one standard for what people find sexy. The standards differ again for what people find beautiful. I've met Playboy Playmates—my friend Diane Stefani worked at one time for the magazine—and they are indeed extraordinary-looking creatures, far beyond the usual specimens, even without airbrushing. The Playboy look, though rare, is certainly an ideal for many men.

But most people hook up for the long haul on compatibility issues—shared worldviews or temperaments. Sex appeal often has little to do with looks; I know several gorgeous men who give off not the faintest whiff of sexuality, and I know men who could crack a camera lens who exude a smutty, irresistible musk.

This was brought home with a sting in *Fat Pig*, an off-Broadway play by Neil LaBute, whose bracing movies (*In the Company of Men, Your Friends & Neighbors, Nurse Betty*) usually explore misanthropy—and misogyny—so extreme it's funny. LaBute is often accused of hating women, and maybe he does and maybe he doesn't, but I find his movies quite the opposite—they satirize the nasty, self-loathing behavior of the worst kind of men, with just enough exaggeration to drive home the offensiveness without taking it out of the realm (and conscience) of the plausible.

In *Fat Pig*, a man finds unexpected bliss with a plus-sized woman who is smart, sexy, and fun and makes him feel the Rocked in a Warm Bath feeling we all crave from a soulmate. The man's vicious coworkers—a conquest-seeking cad and a furious ex-girlfriend in the accounting department—use relentless peer pressure and humiliation tactics to make him doubt himself and reject the great girl who could have made him happy.

The title of the play is purposely provocative. If I hadn't been newly comfortable with the word *fat* by throwing it around each week in my column, I might not have wanted to be seen entering the theater. ("Two tickets for *what?*" "I said *FAT PIG*!!!")

The opening of the play was a fascinating piece of theater in itself. Before the house lights went down, and without any fanfare, the actress playing the—you know, the fat pig—walked onstage with a tray of food and proceeded to eat two (real) slices of pizza. Audience members continued to chat; the couple behind me, after being shushed, protested that the play hadn't started yet—which, of course, it had. (The man who shushed them added, thankfully, "There's an actress on the stage! Have some respect!")

The audience continued to talk while the actress, Ashlie Atkinson, 200 pounds, slowly, deliberately finished those slices. (I have to say I envied her them.) We're talking at least 10 minutes of theater time, during which a large portion of the audience ignored the actress on the stage.

It was a brilliant opening. Fat people, particularly women, are often treated as if invisible. If a gorgeous young thing had walked out on stage, the audience would've been rapt—or maybe just the men, leaving their dates with no one to talk to.

No, I take that back. Men and women both tend to give respect to the favored of society in ways they wouldn't dream of offering those on the fringes. It's a habit that's culturally induced and accepted. I'm surprised anyone brakes for fat people.

And the fat people? Just because we're invisible (or a source of revulsion) to others doesn't mean we're invisible to one another. But we're not necessarily kinder. The fat are cautiously aware of the fat; like double agents, we don't acknowledge one another for fear of wider discovery.

60 POUNDS: DOWNSIZING

Ahhh, there's nothing like the feeling of underwear riding up because it's too big.

As I neared a loss of 60 pounds, I was in a state of perpetual excitement. The changes in my body were an endless source of fascination. I love to feel myself up (not in public, don't worry), but at my heaviest I'd poke and prod out of curiosity to see if I was still there (I was) and still fat (yes). Now I stroked, gazed, marveled. I pranced around like the beauty queen of *Carnival*.

I lost weight everywhere. Old bracelets and watches found their way back to newly slim wrists. The opal ring migrated from pinky to a more suitable finger. Thigh-high fishnet stockings no longer rolled down to puddle at my ankles. No more elastic waistbands. I tightened the bands of my swim goggles; had I lost weight in my face?

Size XL was *way* too big and hung shapelessly. Some Mediums fit better than Large. Airplane seat belts had extra strap left over after being pulled tight across my lap.

I had a lap.

And who knew you could lose weight in your feet? My sneakers went from a men's 10 Wide to a women's 10 Medium, which meant I again had access to pink-and-purple trim if I so desired. All my shoes were flopping off my heels. The only footwear that seemed to fit better were my ski boots, whose red extender hooks would never again be needed. Casualties included the never-worn satin pumps with delicate rhinestone straps. They were too big. They had to go.

Everything had to go. The Housing Works Thrift Shop did very well by me (and the deduction reflected nicely on my tax returns).

Before I lost a single pound, I gritted my teeth and got rid of every single article of clothing that didn't fit at that moment; weight-loss experts say it's an important psychological gesture to show you're ready to deal with your body as it is, not as it might be or used to be. Fat people keep complete wardrobes in every size they ever passed through in hopes they'll pass through again in the other direction on some undefined future date. They also have clothing on retainer from when they were heavier. Those are safety nets; *you never know.*

Instead of Barbie's winter wardrobe or wedding trousseau, it's like Barbie's maternity line—for when she's expecting twins, or triplets, or a small voting district.

All in one groaning closet in which there is, incredibly, nothing to wear.

Discarding all that clothing is terrifying. There's the expense and waste, especially when tags still dangle from items bought on the cusp of a five-pound weight loss that never happened.

Then there's the emotional attachment to special outfits you wore on meaningful occasions. The blue silk dress with pale seashells (size 16) I

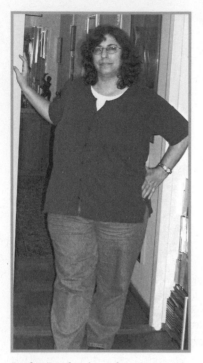

"Before": The day I hit 230 pounds. I saved the pants. *(Photo by Donna Dickman)*

wore when my then-boyfriend's father said he hoped there'd be a wedding in our future. The crisp Calvin Klein skirt (size 10) that quickly went out of style but waited in my closet for some miracle of fashion upheaval. The size 20 denim overalls that were never worn—*what was I thinking?*—but which I couldn't bring myself to part with because that would confirm my temporary insanity. The gorgeous quilted black silk designer jacket (size 2X) I got on sale at the Saks outlet for pennies; what a coup! I wanted to keep it the way hunters keep deer antlers to commemorate their prowess.

The only thing I kept from the old days was the outfit I wore in what became my "before" picture—baggy 3X elastic-waisted blue jeans. I just happened to be wearing them the day I hit 230 pounds. You can see by the look on my face in the photo what I thought of *that*. "I'm going to turn this around," I announced to my friends Donna and Merrick, who were experimenting with their new digital camera, "so you might as well take a picture now." I couldn't manage a smile.

Everyone who loses weight keeps a pair of "fat pants" for those dramatic "after" pictures, and these particular pants were perfect. You can stretch the elastic waist from here to eternity, making it look like you lost more weight than you did. I have a great photo taken by *Daily News* photographer Thomas Monaster at the 50-pound mark. "Stretch them more! More!" he said, snapping away excitedly as if asking Gisele Bundchen to

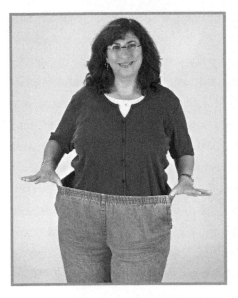 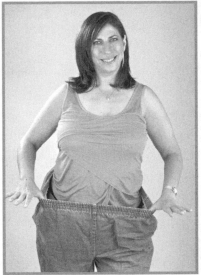

Fat Pants 1: After 30 pounds . . .
(Photo by Thomas Monaster, courtesy
New York Daily News)

Fat Pants 2: After 50 pounds . . .
(Photo by Thomas Monaster, courtesy
New York Daily News)

lick her lips like she meant it. I'm smiling in that photo, but it wasn't because I was happy to lose 50 pounds, it was because I was trying not to
laugh at the efforts Thom and I made to exaggerate the elephantine qualities of the pants. My thumbs were straining so hard to pull them wide I
thought the band would snap.

Getting rid of clothing that doesn't fit involves trust issues. What if you
throw out your "fat" clothes in the belief you'll be successful this time, and
then you aren't? What if you throw out your "thin" clothes as part of the
bargain, keeping only what you can wear so as to stop hedging your bets,
only to find that the psychological ruse works and you lose weight? Either
way, you're screwed. You still have to shell out for a new wardrobe.

It's a leap of faith, also a tautology: If I act as if I believe in myself,
perhaps it will be so.

And it *was* so! I could scarcely believe it. The stupid as-if trick worked! Divesting myself of the clothing and all the baggage it represented acted on me like a tonic. I began losing weight immediately.

It's hard to believe in yourself when it comes to weight loss; faith and fortitude are no match for a sensible blueprint. I believe I can survive in the wilderness because I know I'm perspicacious, a problem solver. Plane goes down? I'd do the Donner Party thing and take a bite out of my seat-mate's buttocks. But weight loss eludes even the most confident and accomplished, because they don't really know how to go about it.

Still I believed—at least enough to get rid of stuff that *did* fit, simply because it didn't look so hot on me. I wasn't just out to lose weight, I was signing on for the whole package—style, fit, quality. The new me. I tried on everything in the closet, with Marie either approving or giving it The Nose. She had a vested interest, since she was still staying on that AeroBed under my home gym and was looking to expand her share of the real estate.

"You have *tons* of closet space!" she'd exclaim.

"I have *no* closet space," I'd say. Every square inch was stuffed with clothing, from T-shirts so tiny they looked like swaddling clothes to the latest addition, the dreaded size 26, which starts to push the outer bounds of the purgatory known as 3X. When I first gained weight, I had no idea there were stores designed just for overweight women; now I was beginning to wonder whether after 3X I might enter a whole new category of specialty store, Omar the Tentmaker or something.

Marie was right. Once I'd carted trunks of stuff to the thrift shop, there was tumbleweed blowing through that closet. Empty hangers tinkled against each other sweetly like wind chimes.

The only downside: What you give to charity can come back to haunt you.

Many years ago I went on a cruise with Amanda. That was the time our friendship nearly ended when she hustled me away from a sizzling, juicy cheeseburger. ("You don't want that," she insisted. *But I do!*" I wailed. I honestly thought I'd strike her.)

Because of Amanda's relentless badgering, we were the only people—perhaps in history—to lose weight on a cruise. We took aerobics classes as the ship listed from side to side. We jogged around the deck every morning with nasty sea spray hitting us in the face. When we docked, the activities director presented the two of us with bright yellow T-shirts that read "I'm shipshape!"

But I wasn't shipshape. I continued to gain weight after the cruise, and the shirt shamed me with its false proclamation. Did I toss it? Of course not! I hoarded it along with all the other clothes I'd never wear. My mother has a phrase for clothing like that—it's for "knocking around the house," meaning, "You'll never wear it, but if you do, make sure no one sees you in it."

Some time after I finally donated the wretched thing to charity, I was walking down the street when a homeless woman headed my way pushing a shopping cart with all her worldly goods, and wearing what could only be my T-shirt. "I'm shipshape!" it crowed. The message was no more incongruous on her than it had been on me.

I was happy to be rid of fashion monstrosities. There are 40 million women over size 14 in America, so you'd think there'd be a lot of great stuff to choose from. But stylish plus-size lines are a relatively recent phenomenon. Most of the larger clothing is still cheap and crappy. *American Demographics* magazine says women spend $25 billion a year on plus-size clothes, and I think all of that $25 billion worth of stuff wound up in my closet at some point.

After it was gone, I didn't miss any of it, not even the satin quilted designer jacket. And I was free to shop for new clothes—within reason, of course. I was hitting a new, smaller size every 15 pounds or so, necessitating yet another high-wire act of faith—as soon as I undergrew a size I immediately shipped out all the barely worn clothes that went with it. I danced in size 18 red satin pants on New Year's Eve, and by January 10 they were in the giveaway pile along with the other 18s. I tried to keep each wardrobe down to a pair of nice pants, a pair of jeans, two skirts, and a few tops.

I didn't spend much. I got a lot of stuff cheap on eBay (and learned the buzzword "NWT"—new with tags). Marie had recently lost 35 pounds and gave me hand-me-downs. Helene began training for a triathlon and her old clothes were fitting her like gunnysacks; she'd leave bags of them on my doorknob. My weight-loss wardrobe of castoffs and found items was, shall we say, eclectic, a mélange of other people's styles and colors. The New Me would have to wait just a little longer.

Getting clear of the plus sizes was like being allowed to stay up till midnight for the first time. The wonders that greeted me! It got so I could hardly wait to toss the "old" stuff—I'd only worn it a few months—and rush to the stores to see what magnificence was available the next size down. Underwear riding up my butt was cause for celebration and a trip to an Ann Taylor outlet where I scored some sweet summer skirts for $10 apiece.

At 57 pounds, I realized—as if for the first time—how great my calves looked. Mere months before, I had been worrying about hemlines that brushed the backs of my thighs and hoping they'd bring back the peasant skirt. But at 57 pounds, nothing longer than mid-thigh would do. A "short" skirt in the Women's department means below the knee—if not blanketing the entire community—but in Misses, short skirts meant business.

Most people think the clothing part of weight loss will be a snap. Who wouldn't want to shop with abandon for a smaller size, a louder color, a trendier style?

Oh, little grasshopper, you have much to learn!

Just because you pine for Scarlett O'Hara's 17-inch waist, "the smallest in three counties" (although it wouldn't have stayed that way if she kept eating everything her suitors brought her at the barbecue), it doesn't mean you can predict the emotional fallout that happens the day you lace that bodice up tight. Helene bequeathed me a sexy wrap-dress that looked spectacular, but it was months before I felt I deserved to wear it. I was still in the fat-person mind-set of trying to blend in, not stand out.

One reader who lost a lot of weight warned that the body never returns to the proportions of your dreams. Your body arrives on Planet Slim as if the molecules got reassembled during transit—see Jeff Goldblum in *The Fly*—with the waist serving as a dividing line between one size for the top, an altogether different size for the bottom.

In Rosie O'Donnell's introduction to Camryn Manheim's book *Wake Up, I'm Fat!,* she writes about the dilemma of "to tuck or not to tuck." Each smaller size requires fresh decisions. As you fit into smaller sizes, the cut, the style, the whole gestalt of the clothing—even the section of the department store in which it's sold—are unfamiliar territory.

As a fat person, I chose clothing out of gratitude at finding something, *anything,* that fit. As I neared 60 pounds, I got picky—lots of trips to the

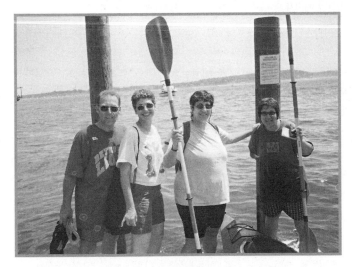

From left: Merrick Bursnk, Donna Dickman, me, and Diane Stefani. I decided to include this photo in the interests of full disclosure. Yes, I was truly fat. *(Photo by Terry Peikin)*

tailor, new conditions that had to be met before I closed the deal. Clothing shopping wasn't a breeze, although it was significantly breezier than at 230 pounds.

I found out the hard way just how nonbreezy it could be when I hit the 60-pound mark. The newspaper suddenly decided we needed new photos. The next day.

I happened to be out of town on a hiking vacation. All I had with me were shorts, T-shirts, hiking boots, and those sport bras that squash you into a mono-bosom. No makeup, no skirt, not even a blow-dryer. Ten pounds before, I'd had my hair and makeup done for the progress photo; this time, the 10-pound milestone was shaping up as a disaster.

⭐ The Makeup Artist

Makeup artist Kian Stave took me to Sephora. This is like having Van Cliburn help you pick out a Steinway. "Too blue . . . too yellow," muttered Kian as she applied creams and sticks and unguents to my face.

With weight loss came a natural desire for a makeover. I'd been using the same palette of colors for years, and meanwhile the cosmetics industry had come up with all kinds of new products—lip stain that plumps and clings, moisturizers that absorb oil and double as foundation, powders that catch the light like Swarovsky crystals.

Kian's father was a painter, and she figures that's how she came by her affinity for working with brushes and mixing colors. In 45 minutes, she taught me how to do the Asiatic eyelash curl, make baby-rabbit eyes, keep my lips moist, and do "smoky" without "raccoon." She wrote down full instructions on how to use my basketful of goodies, then gave me a parting tip: "It's all about the blending."

And it was.

It's no small thing, shopping for One Perfect Outfit. Some women spend a lifetime on it. Although I'd gone from 3X to Large (size 14ish, depending on the cut), it wasn't like I had a world of possibilities at my fingertips. I was still fat, just less so. The only option on such short notice and so far from home base was a nearby mall that catered—as they all do—to teenage girls. Damned if I was going to pose in a top with rhinestone sprinkles spelling out "Hello Kitty."

I bought a complete outfit, plus shoes, makeup, and makeup brushes, in less than two hours. It would have to do. I had particular trouble with the heels, because I wear a European size; don't ask.

The photographer was a local freelancer who shot me upward; ladies over thirty, I think you know what I'm saying.

It was a bad hair day, a bad clothing day, and certainly a bad shoe day. With that photo angle, it was a bad chin day. A bad everything day.

It was to be the last regular Shrinking Critic column. My editors had only agreed to run it for a year, and, fundamentally, they had bought into the very media hype they were guilty of inventing—that you can lose tons of weight overnight and be done with it. The column was taking up prime real estate in the upfront news hole, and there were already grumblings from reporters who covered topics they imagined were more important than my weight loss—like terrorism, global unrest, earthquakes. The column had been a great success with the readers, but I went out on one of the worst photos ever shot of me, wearing hideous clothing that couldn't possibly express the absolute delight I was taking in my new body.

62 POUNDS:
THREE LITTLE EGGS

I thought I had the whole weight-loss thing licked, when a box of Cadbury chocolate eggs humbled me.

I was visiting Marie in London. She bought us a box of three Cadbury Creme Eggs, a popular U.K. treat. Imagine: Chocolate ovals with white creme filling and a touch of orange to suggest yolk. The faintly repulsive ad campaign encourages you to "dip in the goo to release your naughty, playful side!"

In the morning after Marie left for work, the red-blue-yellow box of chocolate eggs chirped to me. Undoubtedly, I thought, I should dip in the goo at least once, since supplies are apparently limited, being available only from January through Easter—or so the marketing strategy claimed, despite annual sales in the U.K. of the equivalent of three eggs per person, 180 calories per egg.

There it was, a rare opportunity combined with a magnetic force field.

Close encounters, indeed. I would eat just one egg. There was even a case to be made for two.

I ate all three. Then I had breakfast.

What did I tell myself as I reached for those eggs? That this is the kind of behavior that made me fat in the first place? That this flies in the face of all my hard work to shed 62 pounds?

No. In a chocolate-induced narcolepsy, full of flavorful overtones of childhood food fortification and a subconscious connection between "eggs" and that lovely, precognitive swim in amniotic fluid, I told myself that this treat was the last of its kind, at least for a year, perhaps forever. The U.K.'s supplies are depleted. Leftovers . . . what are leftovers?

Shame set in. (A stomachache, too.) Forget the National Gallery; I spent the day scouring London for a replacement box so I could fool Marie into thinking I was in control of my chocolate lust. I must have gone to every sweetshop and takeaway counter in that city. The sky darkened. The wind whipped up. I was frantic, perspiring. Marie would be back soon like the mother in *The Cat in the Hat*, and my house wasn't in order.

Cadbury Eggs are so popular in London that they're actually sold from vending machines in the Underground. There it was on the station platform, a red-blue-yellow machine mocking me, mocking me. I ran toward it slo-mo as if in a Breck commercial, arms outstretched toward my beloved. But the machine dispensed only bite-sized mini-eggs, not the full-sized version that had been on Marie's table. It would be like the cuckoo sneaking its eggs into the nests of other birds; Marie would never raise these mini-eggs as her own.

Finally, in a Boots pharmacy, I found foil-wrapped, normal-sized eggs, and it dawned on me that I didn't need a new box of three, I only needed to stuff two individually wrapped eggs in the old box.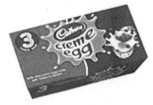

Which I did. And I got away with it. Until I let Marie read this passage in my manuscript. She was so appalled she didn't know what to say.

It's possible to learn new habits. Old ones can be broken. The brain actually generates neurological pathways to accommodate the switch. But those crusty old dendrites from my former habits are still littering my internal landscape—who's responsible for sweeping around here?—because the Cadbury incident occurred after 62 hard-lost pounds. This was the *improved* me, and I was *still* helpless around food.

A weird thing happens when you lose a lot of weight: You get to plateaus, and I don't mean the ones where your body is adjusting and wants to catch its breath before plunging in again. I'm talking about mental plateaus. It's not one joyride down the scale. I remember what was going on at each particular weight when I first hit those numbers on the way up, and as I passed the same numbers on the way down, it was like seeing my life unfold in reverse. Oh—this is what I weighed when my father died. This is what I weighed when I was diagnosed with breast cancer. This is what I weighed when I thought I was going to marry that guy.

Powerful stuff, these memories. Revisiting them is like those murder mysteries where they re-create the scene and it's so evocative that the amnesiac suddenly remembers everything and the killer inadvertently blurts out a confession. The grief over my father's death, the terror of the cancer diagnosis, the utter foolishness of that relationship . . . the scale pricked the scab off those memories and they flooded back in nightmarish detail.

At 60 pounds, I was thrilled, I was dating, I was looking good. And I was scared. With the end of the *Daily News* column, I was no longer committed to losing a pound a week. I hovered at 60 pounds for a long, long time. Months. I seemed perfectly content there, allowing my body to settle into its new dimensions like a house settling into its foundations. Weight maintenance is its own challenge, no less absorbing than weight loss. Sometimes I went up a pound, sometimes down, but I continued eating more or less sensibly, going to the gym four days a week, using the same behavioral tools as before.

When I finally thought I was ready, I cautiously advanced down the scale again, trimming back the calories just a bit, sending a detailed food diary to the Nutrition Twins every now and then so they could kick my tires.

I lost two more pounds.

I realized I might never achieve my original goal—it was becoming clear that 100 pounds was too ambitious and unrealistic a number. But this I knew, with absolute certainty: *I would never gain that weight back again.*

RELAPSE

I gained back 10 pounds.

At *least* 10 pounds; I was afraid to step on the scale and check.

I knew it when my watch, whose excess links I'd so proudly removed, began pinching and angering the flesh of my wrists. At spin class, the irritation from the wristband was so great I'd take off the watch and hang it on the handlebars, hoping against hope that I'd remember to retrieve it. You can make a living entirely from selling watches people have left dangling from the handlebars of Manhattan's spin cycles.

I knew it from my clothing. All the new size 14s that had been getting roomy—I had already been laying in a supply of 12s—now hugged me like those sauna suits designed to squeeze the perspiration out of you. Once again my eyes darted down in alarm and fascination as my belly swelled against the waistband and the spaces between buttons gaped to make way for a chest-bursting alien. The night before I left for Marie's wedding, I frantically went online to order a linen blouse one size up and had it overnighted at an expense nearly equal to the blouse itself.

I knew it from the frequency with which I was eating when I wasn't hungry, all rules broken. Was it "degrees of on" or "degrees of off"? I couldn't remember. I didn't want to remember. The Great Slide had begun, when you leave the land of Unwise, Better, Best for whatever is entombed beneath Unwise. I've been to that place before. It's where you eat without realizing you're chewing, let alone knowing what's on your fork. My reader Irwin is fond of calling food a medication, the kind that people abuse to cover their pain until the day they wake up addicts. Yes, food is a medication—and they sell it over the counter!

⭐ Readers: The One-Stepper

Trudy Trotta of Breezy Point is only half kidding when she says that alcoholics have the advantage. "They need never pick up that glass again. How easy my life would be if I could walk away from food . . . *forever*. Those of us with weight problems are expected to diet yet keep eating. For me it's not one day at a time, it's *one meal* at a time!"

Food is also a deadly weapon, self-mutilation from a shard of chocolate bark.

It wasn't just that I was regaining weight. I was in thrall to food again, worshipping at its well-stocked altar, accompanied by crashing waves of self-loathing. I slumped and scowled through my days, ashamed, angry, depressed, unnerved.

I had nothing to wear.

Had I ever been the Incredible Shrinking Critic? Had I ever known how to lose weight, losing it with relative ease week after week? It must have been a lifetime ago. Now I was in my own private Food Hell.

Here's the difference between people like me who are drawn to disordered eating and people like Marie who happen to gain a few pounds, take note, then lose them: Marie doesn't have reservations under her name for a room in Food Hell, an all-you-can-eat resort where food is both solace and bludgeon, where hopelessness reigns. You don't have to be fat to know this hell; there are thin people here too, anyone who finds it easier to make out their taxes than to resist a slice of pecan pie.

I'll probably struggle all my life to maintain a decent weight. Just because I lost 62 pounds didn't mean I got the Chunky Monkey off my back. I'd achieved a temporary truce that would have to be renegotiated every so often, just like the city's contract with the sanitation workers. Concessions would have to be made. Despite my best efforts, every now and then the trapdoor would open and I'd be whisked back down the chute to Food Hell. Once again I'd crawl through vents and secret passageways in an effort to stay a step ahead of armed security guards who want to keep me there for a nice long stay. Hey, it's not so bad—there's 24-hour room service!

"You divide your time between Bali and Paris? How nice for you! I divide my time between New York and *Food Hell*."

After enough trips to this infernal resort, at least I know where the exits are and, optimally, I can start dragging my sorry self toward them sooner into my stay. *No time for mambo lessons on the Lido deck, thanks. I'm checking out early!*

What sent me careening back to Food Hell with matched luggage and an open-ended ticket?

Oh, so many things.

First, a taxi hit me. Then things *really* got rough.

I wasn't hurt—at least not physically—yet being hit by a cab (in a crosswalk in broad daylight) seemed to let loose the demons of bad karma. Good thing I don't believe in karma, good or bad, because things got so bad that a superstitious person would've had to behead chickens every night in some basement Santeria rite as penance.

The taxi nipped me in the crosswalk, where I had what we pedestrians foolishly call "right of way." The cabbie must have hailed from a country where it's encouraged to make the widest possible turns, because he got me in the middle of a very broad multilane confluence of avenues—they don't call it "Broadway" for nothing—after making such a turn. I spied him from the corner of my eye and automatically broke into an admirably fast run; I mean, I go to the gym! Where I work on "balancing the core" and improving hand-eye coordination and response time!

So I ran. And he rammed me.

I was stunned that a cabbie in my native New York would have the temerity to smash into me, yet my first thought was a happy one—that I was so gosh-darned athletic that I had *just yesterday* bought new running sneakers. The taxi ran over my left foot (I felt the vehicle kind of rise up and plop down on the other side of it), but the sturdy toe box of the new footwear protected me entirely. It was like when that Gristedes super-market that was marked for demolition crumbled on top of a $6,000 baby stroller on the Upper West Side; that Rolls-Royce of strollers closed in like a cocoon and protected the infant just the way my new sneakers snuggled my foot and its more than 100 little muscles, tendons, and ligaments.

But I was pissed. The wheel running over me pinned me in mid-run for a moment, causing my body to slam onto the hood. When I righted myself, I slammed my open palm on the hood—an echo of sorts—to express my displeasure. The driver did what any professional driver and caring human would do in a situation like this: he pretended it didn't happen. He further pretended I wasn't standing there in outrage. He averted his eyes as if I wasn't yelling at him through his windshield. When he finally rolled down the passenger-side window, he said in his defense: "You ran into my car!"

"*Why* would I do that?" I asked indignantly.

"I don't know." He shrugged.

I wish I could say that a kindly cop strolled over to straighten things out. But no cop appeared. No onlookers bestirred themselves from their coffee-shop stools where they watched through a plate-glass window, with their Sunday-morning muffins and double-skinny lattes and peace of mind undisturbed.

There were three solid citizens in the back seat of the taxi, a family of tourists who also looked straight ahead, refusing to acknowledge me or roll down the window. After I frantically made the international symbol for roll it down a crack, which they misinterpreted as the international symbol for please ignore me, I'm just plain nuts, they rolled it down exactly that, a crack, and no further. They appointed one of their tribe as official spokesperson, and after whispering consultation, he declared, "We didn't see anything." Oh, right, of course. They looked on me as a wacky tourist attraction, the kind they were warned about in the guides—"Indigenous population consists of middle-aged women who attempt to hurl themselves in front of cabs in desperate attempts to collect insurance money."

I took the driver's information. I knew I'd be bruised and sore the next day but I wasn't seriously hurt, so I didn't summon help. I had more pressing matters. I was on my way to Costco.

I'm sure I don't need to explain that further. Anyone with a Costco card understands that you don't fritter away precious time getting your skull checked for fractures when you could be buying rolls of bathroom tissue by the caseload.

I took the subway, met J. and his J-mobile, and went shopping for such indispensables as 24-packs of Lean Cuisine and hefty, artificially orange salmon steaks that overflowed their packaging like so many discolored mink stoles. As the day progressed and I loaded my cart with matched sets of sateen bedding and two fire extinguishers "just in case," it became clear that I was having a delayed reaction to the accident.

It was in the parking lot of Pizzeria Uno before lunch when the unpleasant tapeworm of anxiety first slithered through my system and took up residence. For months after, that tapeworm lived it up, pumping icky, inky chemicals through my body—anxiety, fear, feelings of doom and despair.

The taxi incident was just a warning shot over the bow. It reminded me of mortality. I don't know about you, but I just *hate* it when I realize I might, after all, die. I first experienced that sensation when I was being treated for breast cancer. Staring death in the face is like looking at the *Mona Lisa*—it's an awesome spectacle if you can get close enough to see it, but the crowds keep you from catching more than just a brief glimpse, a mere idea of it. Mortality is always there, looming, but we never really look at it except when we get cancer (or a heart attack or a cab runs over our toe). Then it's like getting a private viewing by the museum curator. *Step right this way, Ms. Bernard. I shall pull back the curtain, and there it is—YOUR EVENTUAL DEATH—something you can't do fuck-all about!*

We can any of us die at any moment, from any old thing—a terrorist attack, carelessness, rotten luck. But you don't want to walk around *really* thinking about this. The wisest course is to let lovely denial take over so you don't have to make sure everything you say is well crafted in case it turns out to be your final words.

Being hit randomly by an errant taxi made me unsure of my footing, quite literally. I didn't know where to step. As physically cautious as I am, I can never be sure someone else won't do something crazy with a moving vehicle. Is any place safe? Any route or mode of transportation?

Two days later, while pondering such issues and feeling vulnerable, I had an attack of something—who knows what—and had to check into the ER after all. Raised in a family of alarmists, I went from "It's just a stomachache" to "It's cancer again and I'm dying" within the span of giving the address of the hospital to the cabdriver (a different one, I trust). I got on the cell phone with my sister and my voice immediately took on the querulous tone our mother gets when she's frightened. "I'm sure it's nothing," I said, my voice breaking into a thousand pieces.

Short story long, it was not the internal bleeding that I suspected had occurred from the taxi accident, and it was not cancer. I never say no to morphine—at least I got *something* out of the deal—but I spent the next two weeks going in and out of expensive, degrading tests that never quite proved my internist's theory that the cause was gallstones. His theory suffered from what in my view was a major flaw—my gallbladder had been removed twenty years ago.

"You can still get gallstones," he said flatly, unwilling to abandon his position.

"From where?"

The doctor waved his hand airily, as if to say, Those gallstones, so capricious!

As a lifelong needlephobe, I also had the honor of once again encountering nurses and technicians who confirm my suspicion that when I speak, it is in Aramaic or some other ancient language.

"Wow, you have no veins!" said a male nurse as he poked and prodded.

"Could you please not discuss the quality of my veins? I'm afraid of needles and I don't want to hear anything about my veins."

"Oh, sure. Right. It's just that whoever took your blood last, they sure *blew out your veins.*"

"I don't want to *hear* about it!"

"Yeah, okay. Mum's the word. I'm just saying that *a million things can go wrong with venipuncture.*"

That phrase . . . it echoes hollowly inside me in the dark of night: "A million things can go wrong with venipuncture . . . venipuncture . . . venipuncture . . ."

So now I'd been hit by a cab, which undermined my sense of safety. And I was having costly tests for whatever was sending my liver functions zooming.

Then my breast-cancer surgeon, the woman who saved my life, was mowed down by an ambulance and died.

It happened while she was in the crosswalk of bustling Second Avenue, only half a block from the Memorial Sloan-Kettering cancer clinic, where she worked.

I won't insult her memory with jokes. This was horribly tragic; even my friends who met Jeanne Petrek back when she was caring for me were crying. Petrek was at the forefront of research into the long-term prospects of people like me—women who'd had breast cancer relatively young and who still wanted to bear children. That was only one of her projects, a ten-year study that was just wrapping up when the ambulance—*an ambulance!*—killed her.

I wrote an appreciation of Dr. Petrek for the next day's *Daily News*. The doctor-patient relationship can be very intense; I dedicated my book *Breast Cancer, There & Back* to Petrek and the two other cancer doctors who guided me back to health in 1996. Writing about her for the paper was cathartic but difficult, forcing me back in memory to when mortality wasn't a theoretical concept for me. How many times are they going to give me private viewings of that damn *Mona Lisa?*

Dr. Petrek was hit in a daylit crosswalk, just the way a taxi had hit me a few days earlier. Those events had nothing in common, yet I shivered at the reminder of how lucky I'd been.

The day I wrote on deadline about my doctor, Abu was sneezing. Abu is—well, *was*—Marie's elderly puffball of an Abyssinian cat. The only problem I'd had with taking Abu for six months while Marie was in London was that if something happened to the cat, it would be bad for me, bad for Marie, bad for our friendship. The last thing I wanted was a dying cat on my hands.

The story of Abu's rapid decline—the weird sneezing was really a series of paroxysms set off by internal decay, in turn caused by kidney failure—is a sad one, and still too full of grief for me to tell in full. It involved administering IV fluids under Abu's skin twice a day—not a happy chore for a needlephobe. Abu was a needy cat—you know how I feel about "needy"—but when he was ill, I had him sleep between my legs so I could monitor his labored breathing in the night. That cat had lived to purr—you could actually hear him down the hall from my apartment—but there were to be no more purrs. He wouldn't eat. He seemed confused, staring into his water bowl as if not remembering how to drink. In daily consultation with Marie by phone, I eventually made the decision to take Abu to the vet for his final journey, a decision and an ordeal that was so painful it seemed to damage me in some fundamental way, the horror of it clawing at a dark place inside me.

I don't like to think about Abu anymore. I actively push away the memory of him. I didn't enjoy writing this passage. And when you picked up this book, I'll bet you didn't say, Wow, a book that goes into grueling detail about rocking and cuddling a cat into death! A must-read!

Taxi, emergency room, doctor, cat . . . it all happened in the span of

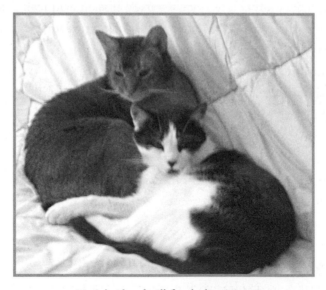

Marie's Abu, the ill-fated Abyssinian,
and my Buzz, who adored him.

two weeks. I was desolate, angry, also numb. Let's see if I've got it straight: Life is short, the body is frail, and no matter what decisions I make there are unspeakable repercussions.

I started to cry. A lot. I'd burst into tears for no apparent reason. I called Marianne, trying to sound offhand, to see if she wanted to meet me for dinner at the Greek place. The minute she sat down, I wailed myself into hiccups. I was so . . . *needy.*

I did the only logical thing: I put my apartment on the market. *Because there just wasn't enough stress in my life.*

I spoke to a real-estate broker on a Monday, held an open house that Sunday, sold it the following day for $150,000 over the asking price. (It was a great, great apartment, and Ann's a great broker.) Then, despite vowing to rent instead of rushing back into the superheated housing market, I bought a condo that wasn't yet built. *Because there wasn't enough stress in my life.*

I'd get up, go to the gym, write some reviews. Around 3 P.M., the anxiety would start leaking from every pore, a hissing acid leak that sizzled everything it touched. I'd curl up in a ball, neither sleeping nor relaxing, palpitating with anxiety and dread. Must get a grip. Must lose weight. Must put one foot in front of the other.

My to-do list was so long it was like one of those cartoon scrolls that roll out forever when the trumpeter reads a message at the king's court. Figure out where to live for ten months between apartments. Sell furniture I never liked anyway. Send change-of-address cards to 1,450 contacts in Rolodex. Pack. Lose weight. Write weight-loss book. Act normal.

Surely I wasn't the first person to feel sick and drowning in anxiety. What do the others do? "They drink!" said my friend Linda, who knows what she's talking about.

Of *course!* Why didn't I think of that?

I like a nice cold martini every so often, mostly for the drunken, fleshy olives. But alcohol has lost much of its appeal for me over the years. And recreational drugs are so unattractive in people over thirty. What to do, what to do . . .

Ah, yes. I'll *eat!* Food never disappoints.

I'd learned *nothing.* Or maybe I'd learned that, all bad habits considered, food as comfort isn't the worst. Already shocked, distressed, and vulnerable, I saw food as a reasonable crutch to get me through the packing, moving, deadlines. It would obscure my memories of holding Abu steady on the vet's table. It would soothe me like the love of Heathcliff from beyond the grave.

I didn't go wild. I was still striving for low-fat over high, still meeting Diane Stefani at the gym three to five times a week—grimly, for sure, but consistently. My body still felt sleek and powerful. But the eating was out of control again, and it was a double misery—*I'm getting fat and I'm writing a book on losing weight, for chrissake!*

Pulling back in the middle of a binge is immensely difficult. I wasn't technically in a binge—it's not like I was surrounded by desserts of many nations—but my whole mind-set had regressed. I was back in precontemplation. I needed help.

If there's one thing I recommend above all else when you're being burned alive in Food Hell, it's asking for help. Don't be proud, be practical.

I e-mailed the Nutrition Twins. They responded like EMTs, ambulance lights flashing, sirens blaring.

First, I had to report to them everything I ate. Accountability makes a difference—not only are you admitting to yourself what you're doing, but other eyes are on you too.

Using sensitive micro-instruments, the Twins were able to detect a morsel of hope among the salty Frito crumbs. They noticed I was still trying for grilled fish or chicken, even if I was supplementing meals with lemon-iced pound cake at Starbucks.

"Why not try Cheerios and skim milk and a banana tomorrow morning?" suggested Tammy. Or maybe it was Lyssie.

The next day dawned bright and beautiful. I had a black-and-white cookie.

The cookie wasn't rewarding. It was the *idea* of a black-and-white cookie that I was after, a memory of childhood treats with my father. There must exist somewhere a genuine black-and-white cookie that meets the standards of my nostalgic reverie: Cakey, with a moist yin-yang topping that doesn't peel off like a dried facial mask. The cookie I ate was not that cookie. I couldn't recapture childhood, or Daddy, with this trans-fat, assembly-line junk food.

The second morning dawned bright and beautiful. I had Cheerios.

Success breeds success. For lunch I had hummus on toasted whole-wheat pita. I felt like the Wright Brothers when the engine finally turned over. I had an early dinner of steamed vegetables with steamed chicken from a Chinese takeout place. It was a perfect food day.

But it wasn't over.

My gym buddy, Diane, and her husband, Terry—a chef—had taken me in during my hiatus between apartments. I split my time between their house and Marie's guest room. I finished my healthy dinner of steamed vegetables and chicken, took the train back to Queens, walked in the door, and found that Terry had cooked up a huge batch of salmon, rice, and beans.

"We waited for you!" Diane sang out, looking relieved that I'd finally arrived.

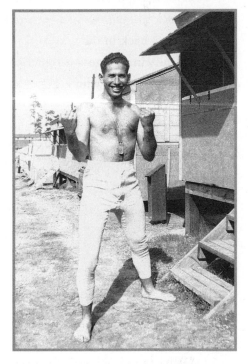

Daddy stationed in the Pacific in WWII. Eating black-and-white cookies won't bring him back.

127

Gulp.

They'd delayed their own dinner for hours to accommodate me, gone to great lengths to please me and make me feel welcome. I didn't have the heart to tell them I'd already eaten.

Plus, an overeater doesn't turn down a meal. Certainly not a meal prepared by a chef.

I ate a second dinner.

Still, the day was a success. Terry's dinner was one of life's many unanticipated (and this time, pleasurable) events. You can't regiment every bite you put in your mouth. I had tried, done my best, pulled myself back from the brink; that's what counted.

The next couple of weeks went easier. The insane eating subsided. The swelling in my wrist went down so my watch didn't rub. Some of those extra 10 pounds had been water weight after all. It was not a disaster, not the end of my life or proof that I'm hopeless. The occasional setback—even a dramatic relapse—is an inescapable part of the journey of weight loss.

Moral of the story:

- When you find yourself on a return trip to Food Hell—and you will—look for the exit vents and secret passageways; you know where they are.
- Always call ahead and let Diane and Terry know your dinner plans.

★

Terry asked me later: "Why did you gain that weight back?"

"Stress," I said.

"No, really, why did you gain it back?"

Diane and I both looked at him. "You're kidding, right?" asked Diane.

Terry is another of that breed that just doesn't get it, doesn't understand the psychology of overeating. As a chef, he's around food all day and it doesn't have a hold on him. I've seen him prepare a meal and walk away, distracted, as if he somehow forgot there's a giant plate of steaming succulence right there. That's something that's not likely to happen to me.

When Terry asked why I'd gained weight back, what he wanted was an answer he could understand: "I ate."

Yes, I ate. It's calories, ultimately, that are responsible for weight gain—but only in the strictest sense, because food is neutral, neither good nor bad. It's the *behavior* that creates a problem.

Beyond that, stress really does contribute to weight gain, right down to the chemistry of it. When under stress, we experience the fight-or-flight syndrome, a physical response that slows digestion and pours adrenaline through the system. Our bodies are designed so if a wildebeest is attacking, we're primed to sink a spear in its gut or else run like the wind.

For that we need energy and tension. The body supplies it; here comes the adrenaline, followed closely by the increase in heart rate. You're tense, you're vigilant, the blood pressure spikes, your pupils dilate so you can catch the wildebeest's every move.

What else do you need in this situation? A plate and fork, obviously, for the wildebeest dinner you'll be enjoying later around the campfire. But first you need to fuel that energy . . . *with food!* Particularly with carbs, because that's the fuel of choice for action. (When you exercise, especially at high intensity, your muscles burn off sugar, or carbohydrate, before looking around for something else to throw in the furnace.)

The body under stress conditions also sends a lovely hit of cortisol, a steroid hormone from the adrenal gland that makes you hungry and helps you store fat. Cortisol is an interior decorator: *I envision a wall of FAT over here, with a walk-in closet for FAT over there . . . Oh, here's a delivery of FAT, I must sign for that!*

But, you argue, the wildebeest *didn't* attack. In fact, you're not sure what a wildebeest is; do they carry it at Whole Foods? And, on further inspection, it turns out the wildebeest is a vegetarian and its worst offense is that it rolls in its own excrement, so it's more likely to offend you to death than gore you.

Doesn't matter. Your body doesn't know the difference. When there's stress, the body is *positive* it's another wildebeest, it's programmed that way, that's all there is to it. You can't call up the autonomic nervous system on the house phone and say, "Hello? Is this my autonomic nervous system? Sympathetic division? I just want to clarify that the stress out here is that *I'm late for my train.* No, no, not a wildebeest at all. False alarm. So could you hold off on the cortisol and turn down the adrenaline pumps a bit? They're clanging in my head."

You don't have that choice. The autonomic nervous system won't take your call.

Sick cat? Fight-or-flight response, get Devil Dogs, stat! Selling your house? Fight-or-flight response, need Twinkies on the double! Weird living arrangement, crushing deadlines, things not going your way? Send in more fat, need more fat!

Psychologist Howard Rankin likes to quote the Woody Allen line "I've had many problems in my life and some of them have actually happened." Anxiety is worrying about what *might* happen. Maybe *nothing* will happen. Probably a wildebeest *won't* eat you. But it's too late—you've rung the stress bell, the body's gears are turning, and for the millionth time chemicals are flooding your system, demanding attention.

Those chemicals have a lot to say about how we eat. Fat people often don't know what real hunger feels like. Perhaps they've ignored or lost touch with their body's chemical signals. That's the trouble with the overly simplistic "just eat less" or "eat when you're hungry, stop when you're not" philosophies. Sure—if you're reading the signals right to begin with.

Studies have found that sometimes—particularly when you don't get enough sleep—the body's supplies of leptin are low. The hormone leptin is the chemical trigger that, when it sees food pouring in, rushes to the hypothalamus and begs it to turn off the hunger spigot. It takes about 20 minutes from the time your body has had enough to eat for the hormone leptin to make the big announcement upstairs and for the press releases to go out—which is why if you can stop eating somewhat sooner than usual, the hunger urge is likely to dissipate as the leptin catches up.

But not always. Not in people who didn't get enough sleep, for example. And those people are known to have a tendency to gain weight. Leptin (whose name derives from *leptos,* meaning "thin") takes its sweet time in fat people, probably because there's not enough of it. The "I'm full" signal reaches the hypothalamus late, and shyly. It's a chicken-egg thing: Do fat people overstimulate their leptin until it pops its cork and lies broken and moaning in some dark alley of the body? Or do people with faulty leptin production get fat because there's no Jiminy Cricket hormone to tell them to put the fork down?

Jeffrey Friedman at Rockefeller University first discovered leptin in 1994. It was the beginning of looking at fat not as a collection of billions of tiny, overstuffed bladders but as an endocrine organ all its own. I see a horror movie in the making: *It's a bird! It's a plane! No . . . it's my fat! And it wants revenge!*

Leptin was an early star in the research into the chemical component of appetite. It's what decides on your behalf during a diet that what you're really trying to do is pull a palace coup and starve yourself to death. In response, your metabolism slows, so much so that you can actually experience the side effects of malnutrition, including fatigue and irritability. And that could put you in danger of defying the maxim that fat people are jolly.

Then, when you eat again, your body banks a little extra fat; *you never know . . .*

Leptin problems can begin in infancy, programming certain individuals to eat more. That doesn't mean you *have* to eat more, just like if you're in a bank and they leave the money out, you don't *have* to stuff it in your bag and flee. But certainly the temptation is there. Malfunctioning leptin leaves you ravenous, fighting off feelings of starvation, while those folks with their perfect leptin-producing systems assume everyone feels the way *they* feel, untroubled by the siren call of food. Since *they* feel full after eating just a little—the smug bastards—they assume fat people must feel the same way and are just being obtuse, as well as obese. (See? I said the "o" word! But only in pursuit of a punch line.)

Leptin has since been joined by the discovery of a growing number of chemical triggers that explain how hunger and satiety function (or malfunction) in individuals. They sound like the Seven Dwarfs, or at least some of them: For example, there's ghrelin, an appetite stimulator. People who don't get a full night's rest wake up with too much ghrelin, too little leptin. And just as this book was going to press, obestatin came out like a debutante to an array of admiring suitors. This hormone, discovered at Stanford University, makes you lose your appetite. In mice, anyway. "No more cheese," they squeak, and I'd like to see the day I say what those mice are saying.

You can see where all this research is going—there'll be a day not too far off when hormone therapy will be used to artificially regulate appetite.

These hormones don't let fat people off the hook. When you step back from responsibility and say, "The Devil Dog made me do it," you're not being honest. I don't overeat only because I'm hungry. My eating habits left the land of hunger cues long ago and have soared aloft for years on a current of emotional need and oblivion. Getting my hunger hormones back in sync will no doubt be helpful, but it isn't the whole answer.

Back in my mid-thirties, when I first hit 145 pounds (which seemed intolerable at the time), I went to a seminar given by a nutritional behaviorist. The woman asked the group when the last time was that we'd felt hunger. There were the usual jokes—"Five minutes ago!" "Right now!"

"I can't remember what it's like to feel hungry," I said. "I don't know what hunger is."

At that point in my life, "hunger" wasn't a physical sensation. I was hungry emotionally, sure. Like a ventriloquist's dummy, my emotional needs spoke on my behalf, ordering the waitstaff around: *Give me more, more, more!*

Most of the people in the group felt the same way. Hunger had ceased to be a biological cue and was instead a nagging, constant sensation, a panic and a clenching of the stomach. Hunger to us was the *anticipation* of hunger.

Similarly, we didn't know what it was like to have eaten enough. We never stopped at an appropriate juncture. We knew "full," not "no longer hungry." Only later could I see that the familiar feeling I associated with the end of a meal was actually pain. Ideally, eating shouldn't hurt, yet it did. I assumed that's what you're supposed to feel when you push away from the table: stuffed.

The first exercise in that seminar was to experience actual hunger, to "sit with it" and see how it felt.

It felt *bad*.

The idea was to get back in touch with natural bodily signals, and to observe without judgment the emotional signals that were messing with our heads. Along with rising hunger came rising panic: *I don't know where my next meal is coming from!* Hunger aroused feelings more uncomfortable than the physical heaviness of Thanksgiving dinner with all the trimmings. That's where the real pain was coming from—the emotional trimmings. And that's why we ate, early and often, not because we'd misinterpreted the hunger pangs (although we had), but because "sitting with our feelings" (to use the self-help lingo) was too distressing. We escaped doubt and fear by smothering it in food. We used food to protect us from the very thing the nutritionist wanted us to try—sitting with our feelings, *feeling* our feelings.

What a drag. I hated my feelings. As for experiencing biological hunger, we didn't know then about leptin and hormones, or whether we lacked the appropriate cease-and-desist cues other people were privy to.

A complementary exercise required us to experience the gradual stages of satiety. We'd rate our hunger *and* our fullness on various scales, and it was always the same thing: ravenous hunger filled us with dread, but so did feelings of normal fullness. We wanted to be extra-full, just to make sure.

Actually, it was difficult to test what it was like to be ravenous because none of us wanted to be there. We'd get desperate and halt the experiment for a snack break. We couldn't pretend to be impartial observers in the field; we'd learned the hard way that ravenous hunger was the wolf that picked off the stragglers. Allowing that kind of hunger had annoying repercussions too, because to make up for the experience of it, we were more likely to remain at the table after everyone else was done. When I allow myself to get too hungry, it's a long, dreary night of yo-yo behavior ahead.

The idea back then, before research into leptin and other appetite-regulating hormones and chemicals, was that simply by being attuned to the body's cues you could regain mastery. Can leptin and ghrelin and obestatin be retrained? Can I get seconds on them? I'm assuming, or hoping, that the answer is yes. I imagine that if you can get your body up and running properly with a steady diet of exercise, proper nutrition, and enough rest, leptin production can normalize just as you can normalize certain other facets of blood chemistry. After all, it's easy to adjust to healthy menus; at spas, I quickly and happily embrace the schedule and taste of low-cal meals, relaxing into the routine of them, even welcoming the restrictions. I don't feel forever damned to overeating. But I do feel highly susceptible.

According to *Science News Digest for Physicians and Scientists,* there will be leptin gene therapy in the not so distant future. Sign me up for the beta.

The leptin findings put a major crimp in the claims of the know-it-alls who think fat people should simply pull themselves up by their bootstraps. It's not so easy to push your plate away if you're in a constant state of biologically influenced hunger. To turn your back on food against the advice of your primordial survival instinct is a major feat. Fatphobes with bullhorns (*Just eat less, you sissies!*) might not have a leptin-free memory from which to draw a comparison between their eating behavior and ours. People have no patience for things they've never experienced. "I've never been sold into sexual slavery—but, hey, how bad could it be? Cheer up!"

"Explore your hunger" exercises are worthwhile, no matter your biological predicament. I now know absolutely the difference between "mouth hunger," where you want food for reasons other than nutrition, and "stomach hunger," where your body craves a tank full of gas so it can go racing on the drag strip of life.

A few months after that nutritionist's class, I ran into the teacher downtown. She seemed astonished at how good I looked. It was the gloaming when for a brief, shining moment, I had dieted down to 126, within a measly pound of the *goal du jour*. The nutritionist seemed skeptical, and I can't blame her; she knew I hadn't addressed the underlying issues, so it wasn't likely the pounds would stay off.

For the moment it was all mine, everything I thought I wanted: I was thin, I was hot. But like Orpheus turning back as he was leading Eurydice out of the shades of Hades, I looked back too soon. I thought in my triumph that I was immune, so I had a little snack. The weight came back, and I lost everything.

Again, I'm not trying to shift the blame. My friend Charley said there's nothing less honest than a "Duncan Hines stole my sense of self" memoir. I'm not like Suzanne Somers, who in *Suzanne Somers' Eat, Cheat, and Melt the Fat Away* gives you the benefit of her many years as a research scientist: "If you learn nothing else from this book, I hope you realize that

⭐ Celebrity Eating Disorders

According to the website Caring On Line (www.caringonline.com), celebrities who have come out about their eating disorders include Jane Fonda, Sally Field, Jamie-Lynn Sigler, Victoria Beckham, Justine Bateman, Joan Rivers, Sandra Dee, Mary-Kate Olsen (who has been photographed next to her "eating coach"), Karen Carpenter (who famously died of heart failure after a long struggle with anorexia), Princess Diana, Oprah Winfrey, Elton John, Paula Abdul, Christina Ricci, Billy Bob Thornton, Melanie Griffith, and Janet Jackson.

calories and fat do not cause weight gain. Hormonal imbalance causes weight gain."

There *is* such a thing as hormonal imbalance, and it certainly makes it harder to lose weight. But according to the *Mayo Clinic Health Letter*, "Less than 2 percent of all cases of obesity can be traced to a metabolic disorder or hormonal imbalances."

When I overeat these days, it's a choice. Not a good one. But I'm not saying, "I can't help being fat," only that I have trouble managing my behavior around food.

There are many forces at work when you gain weight—psychological, physiological, circumstantial. Alcohol stimulates appetite while weakening resolve, so the minute you order a drink you're already in trouble, and not just from the empty calories in your glass. The mounting evidence on sleep deprivation points to hormonal fluctuation and carb craving. Childhood soda drinking leads to later weight problems.

Anxiety in children has been linked to eating disorders. Why are they anxious? Another study found that anxious mothers bathe their unborn children in a soup of anxiety that the kids take with them through life. Now there's a good reason to blame Mom!

You don't need multimillion-dollar studies to tell you there's danger lurking in food courts across America: A slice of cheesecake at the Cheesecake Factory can run you 2000 calories, more than a full day's allotment.

"I ate too much" is true. But it's way too simplistic, even meaningless, against the full sweep of the overeating conundrum. Why did I relapse? A taxi, a cat, fear, complacency, leptin, adrenaline, cortisol, everything, nothing.

And food. But somehow, that was the least of it.

★

Here, let's imagine a fantastic voyage inside my brain. We're in search of the wiring to see what happens when I overeat.

Here we are inside my brain. (And it's so big!) Here's the center for eating, which is the offspring of the pleasure and survival centers. There are special sensors here for chocolate, ice cream, and . . . mashed turnips? Pretend you didn't see that.

Right next to the eating center is the one that controls reason. It's humming along, computing calories and processing nutritional tidbits from the latest issue of *Prevention*.

Unfortunately, the two centers aren't plugged into each other. They're like the FBI and the CIA used to be—they refuse to share information! I eat, and no bells go off signifying the eventual consequence of weight gain. Where's the leptin? It's in the coat closet with the new intern.

Mindful eating is something that doesn't come naturally to me. To stay on top of weight loss, you've got to give careful thought to everything you eat: What's it made of? (Is it mostly protein, for repairing muscle?) Am I really hungry? What else is going on in my life that's affecting what

I'm eating? The cheeseburger I wanted so badly on that long-ago cruise with Amanda just happened to coincide with a creeping (and correct) suspicion that my clothes were all wrong, that I wasn't looking good. Quick fix? A cheeseburger.

Mindfulness, like anything else, can become a habit if you reinforce those new neural connections with practice. Even so, sometimes you need to trot out the big guns from your weight-loss arsenal.

An idea occurred to me while reading *The Thin Commandments Diet,* by Stephen Gullo. It's quite an annoying book. The word *powerful* is very powerful to Gullo; every time he describes a method or offers a tip, you can be sure it's a powerful one. When he reveals that his clients cough up $1,000 an hour for his authoritative help and have to wait months for the opportunity to do so, I start to feel about Gullo the way I do about Mireille Guiliano, author of *French Women Don't Get Fat,* who makes her own yogurt from scratch. These two are far too smug for their own good.

What's additionally annoying about Gullo is that I have to pass his office if the elevator is out of service when I stop in at my behaviorist, Stephen Josephson. As I huff and puff past Gullo's more accessible digs, I can almost see the sign: If You Were Willing to Pay $1,000 an Hour, You'd Be Home Now. Josephson's rates are no picnic either, but nothing like Gullo's. Maybe the two of them purposely stall the elevator so their fat patients can get some exercise.

Gullo doesn't look at fat people as losers or moral delinquents (surely not when they're paying him $1,000 a pop), and he offers solid science to back up the mantra "Strategy is stronger than willpower." Gullo dispenses practical behavior-mod advice, most of which boils down to planning ahead and analyzing what you're doing. He doesn't recommend much more than what common sense should tell you—keep a snack handy in case of an afternoon blood-sugar dip, keep a food diary. I especially liked "Plan to avoid trouble," because there's really no reason to "just look" at a dessert menu or stroll by the frozen-foods section on your way to pick up a container of skim milk.

Annoying though he is, Gullo offers sane—maybe even *powerful*—advice. While reading him, I suddenly entertained a revolutionary idea, one I'd previously dismissed many times as sheer insanity.

I decided to give up chocolate and ice cream. Entirely. Not even as an occasional treat.

I decided on a Sunday, and with few exceptions, I haven't touched chocolate or ice cream since. (There was an ugly incident in Zermatt with some chocolates shaped like little Matterhorns, with clever white-chocolate snow peaks and liquored fillings, but the authorities let me go.)

Is it possible, even desirable, to give up foods you adore? Mere seconds before reading the chapter in Gullo's book, I would have argued no, you shouldn't take away the foods that give a person the most pleasure. I'm with the French Women on this one—savor the finest food but in moderation, preferably at an outdoor café in the heart of Paris.

But Gullo makes a good point, one that's nearly as incendiary as the comments Harvard president Lawrence Summers made about women not having a gift for science: There are some people—*people like me*—who can't handle moderation.

For me, there's no such thing as taking it easy, not when it comes to certain very specific trigger foods. We all scream for ice cream—only some of us scream louder. You can keep your beer and potato chips and salted nuts. And though I'm crazy about pasta and cheese, they don't control my life.

Chocolate and ice cream are different. I'm Renfield to their Count Dracula, Igor to their Dr. Frankenstein. *Yes, master, I will bring you corpses from the morgue.*

Experience has shown that "just this once" and every possible trick of portion control or casting the food as a rare treat doesn't work for me

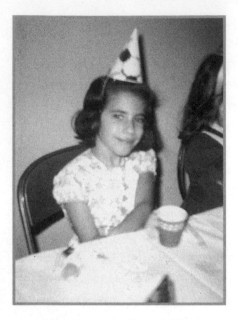

when it comes to chocolate and ice cream. Perhaps some childhood birthday party traumatized me, and like a Nam flashback, I wake up screaming, convinced I have a conical party hat perched on my head.

I can't explain it. And I'm not going back for eighteen more years of talk therapy to get to the root of it. I just want a breather from the tyranny of chocolate and ice cream.

Gullo suggests (studies back him up) that uniquely individual cravings are mostly a matter of neurobiology, not lack of willpower. He cites a home test to see how sensitive you are to the pleasures of taste, using just a pinch of saccharin on the tip of your tongue. If it tastes sweet, you're probably a nontaster. If bitter, you're a supertaster.

Dare I call it a powerful tool?

Like fingerprints and snowflakes, no two tongues are alike. Maybe you got the looks and the smarts, but your tongue was shortchanged on the taste buds. Those with fewer taste buds are harder to satisfy, so they tend to load up on sugary and salty snacks, always looking for the kick that the supertasters get with just a spoonful. The tongues of supertasters are abloom with taste buds, so they get a quick, satisfying rush from treats and don't seem to crave more.

I'd like to put a little saccharin on Mireille Guiliano's tongue, just for fun! And also to confirm what I suspect: that the *French Women Don't Get Fat* author is a supertaster who can live with one flaky pastry a week. Like the gentle movie monster who goes insane when a villager pokes a torch in his direction—*fire makes him crazy!*—you can't give me a little baglet of M&M's or a soupçon of someone's espresso-chip ice cream and there-after expect peace in the neighborhood. It just sets me off.

I'm well aware that M&M's aren't made from the finest chocolate and therefore don't satisfy my philosophy of eating only the finest foods. But there's something about the crunch, the marble-like mouthfeel, the melted ooze from betwixt the cracks of sugar casings. Maybe not today, maybe not tomorrow, but within a week of eating a few M&M's, the taste-and-tactile memory will awaken a part of my brain—a sleeper cell—to seek them out again. When I eat chocolate and ice cream, there is no satisfactory finish.

So why start?

The more I stay away from trigger foods, the more the urge to repeat the experience quiets down. While reading Gullo's book, I realized for the first time in my life that I sincerely didn't want to inflame those urges again. I was tired of the endless loop of anxious eating and unbidden cravings. The drama queen in me liked the idea of the grand gesture—like the time I went totally vegan for six months. What's not to love in a crown of thorns?

I read the Gullo chapter on a Saturday night while finishing off the last of Terry's espresso-chip ice cream. He and Diane were away for the weekend, so I was scavenging Terry's ice cream just as I did in the old days when Marie moved into my place with her luggage of Ben & Jerry's.

The next morning I examined my options: I could buy a replacement gallon and eat it down to the point at which Terry had left off (the Cadbury Egg Option). Or I could apologize to Terry and just give up chocolate and ice cream completely (the Gullo Option).

I went with the advice from the guy who overcharges.

I renounced my worst trigger foods. I wasn't necessarily saying "for-ever," only that these foods were off-limits to me right now and for the foreseeable future. I can always reassess, but, judging by the chocolate Matterhorns in Switzerland, it's still too early.

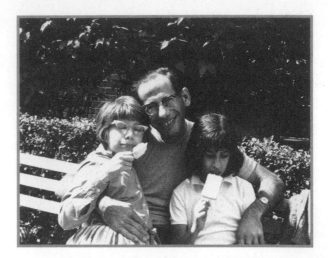

Diane (left), Daddy, and me. Ice cream = love.
(Photo by Gloria Bernard)

If you're reading this book for hints on losing weight, please don't think I recommend giving up your favorite foods. I've been refining my eating habits for a few years, tweaking and realigning as I go along. What seems possible—or desirable—to me now was unthinkable back when I started. Once my friend Helene saw she could do a mini-triathlon, she took the "mini" out and started training for the big leagues; you can't see or consider the next peak until you've climbed the first hill.

I know plenty of overeaters who manage to reserve their trigger foods for special occasions or to enjoy as small, supervised treats without having to make the sign of the cross every time they pass a cookie. It just doesn't work for me.

After my grand gesture, Terry and Diane felt safe in restocking foods I would have killed for at one time. I didn't touch them. Quite frankly, it was a relief. I was relieved of the choice, the struggle. They left packs of M&M's carelessly on the counter; I never salivated. Marie and George had a Ziploc baggie of fine chocolates in the refrigerator; I never un-zipped.

For the first time in my life, my worst trigger foods felt neutral.

My reader Irwin had been e-yelling about this for ages: *Give up sugar!* I thought he was a nutcase. Sometimes you're not ready to see that the bum on the street is really the Sufi master you've been seeking.

70 POUNDS:
WHAT I ATE

A little cottage cheese.

That's what my grandmother would say whenever she'd start one of her frequent recitations of what she ate on any particular day. "A little cottage cheese" became a code phrase my sister and I used to set off tales of Grandma's amusing quirks. She had several pairs of glasses dangling from her neck at all times, one pair for dialing the phone, another for reading, a third for watching TV; we were afraid she'd garrote herself on the cords and lanyards. She believed that a melted cheese sandwich was made by pressing a slice of individually wrapped American cheese, hard and cold from the refrigerator, firmly between the bookends of two burnt pieces of toast. And she was always "on a diet," a mysterious one of her own devising; I hope this book is not some bizarre genetic inheritance from her.

Grandma would get up creakily from her rocking chair, balance unsteadily as if at a podium to deliver the keynote speech, and launch into an enthusiastic rundown of everything she'd had that week, a menu plan whose cornerstone was invariably "a little cottage cheese."

There's nothing more boring than hearing what someone else ate. And yet people keep asking me what I'm *eating* if I'm not following Atkins or Jenny Craig or the Rotation Diet (which really did involve cottage cheese).

So at the risk of sounding like Grandma Gussie, here is what I eat:

A little cottage cheese.

Just kidding, although Friendship makes a spreadable low-fat "whipped" cottage cheese with 1% milkfat that is particularly creamy and goes well with cantaloupe or fresh pineapple. (Avoid canned fruits; they're usually swimming in sweetened syrup. Besides, they're revolting.)

Here's what I might eat on a perfect food day, one in which I'm near the top end of "degrees of on," one in which I have my choice of foods and have anticipated contingencies:

- Before the gym (6 A.M.): Coffee with skim milk, and if there's time, oatmeal with cinnamon and fresh strawberries and banana. (No sugar or butter added. If it's flavored oatmeal, I pour it through a sifter to remove extra sugar.)
- After the gym (8:30 A.M.): low-fat yogurt with Grape-Nuts mixed in for crunch. I've already had a liter of water during and after the workout, but I might have more coffee now or an interestingly flavored tea.
- Late morning (11 A.M.): If I didn't have yogurt earlier. I'll have a combination snack, something to grab-'n'-go that includes protein—such as a mini-Babybel cheese along with the second half of the banana from the oatmeal. (I call this a "snackette." HHHI calls it a "Metabo Meal." Stephen Gullo calls it a "Thin-Pack" and prescribes GG Scandinavian bran crispbread for fiber and taste, to be packed in a Ziploc along with cheese and an apple.)

- Lunch (around 1 P.M.): Turkey breast (fresh off the bone, if possible), tomato, and interestingly flavored or textured mustard on whole-wheat toast. Or hummus with tomato in toasted whole-wheat mini-pita. Or (my favorite) seared tofu over brown rice or steamed vegetables. Or—yes!—*a little cottage cheese* and fresh fruit topped with almond slivers. (I like the almonds toasted, although you lose some nutrients that way.) A side salad with a blend of colors and textures is optimal, dressed with a tiny bit of oil and an interesting balsamic vinegar, like fig, plus something for crunch, like water chestnuts, almond slivers, walnuts, or Grape-Nuts. Sometimes I add parmesan cheese.
- Late afternoon snackette (around 5 P.M., or between screenings): Some variation on the morning snackette, pairing an ounce or less of protein with something else. If I haven't been to the gym, or if I'm not truly flagging in energy, I might skip some or all of the snack.
- Dinner (around 8 P.M.): Broiled salmon with lemon, a half-cup of brown rice, roasted vegetables. Or sushi (or sashimi), miso soup, and salad. Or pasta with grilled chicken, marinara sauce, vegetables, grated parmesan.
- Late-night snackette (around 11 P.M.): Fruit-juice ice pop (15 calories).

★ Chef Terry's Seared Tofu

A satisfying, change-of-pace protein to drape over brown rice, steamed vegetables, or salad: "I marinate firm tofu in ponzu and tamari. (Ponzu is a Japanese citrus vinegar/soy liquid. Tamari is a lighter soy with a less salty flavor.) Then I dredge it in rice flour and sear it in a tiny bit of sesame oil, or just grill it."

I'm not saying I never eat steak or bread. The only foods I've cut out of my repertoire altogether are the trigger foods ice cream and chocolate. I avoid anything fried, and I don't put too many starchy items on the plate at once (corn on the cob shouldn't share space with pasta, for example).

MARIE'S QUESADILLA FOR ONE

Marie calculates her quesadilla as six "points." "The key is to use modest amounts of cheese, a high-fiber tortilla, and lots of low-fat/low-cal flavor."

SERVES 1 GENEROUSLY

One teaspoon oil
2 thin slices red onion, diced
½ zucchini, sliced (You can add other vegetables for flavor, such as diced
    green peppers or tomatillos)
Smoky hot sauce
Mexican salsa (green tomatillo salsa is my favorite)
4 to 5 shiitake mushrooms or 5 to 6 crimini mushrooms, sliced
Chili powder
2 small or 1 large whole-wheat tortilla
1 to 1 ½ ounces shredded cheese (Monterey Jack, Jalapeño Jack, goat cheese,
    or cheddar)

Heat the oil in large nonstick pan or griddle over medium heat. Add the onions and sauté for about a minute, until hot but not softened. Add the sliced zucchini, stirring. Add 4 or 5 drops hot sauce, plus a bit of salsa if more liquid is needed. Add the mushrooms as the zucchini starts to brown. Dust the chili powder over mushrooms. Cook until the mushrooms soften and start to release liquid. Spoon the mixture onto a plate—cover to keep warm.

(continued)

Place the tortilla in the same pan and heat for 1 to 2 minutes. Flip the tortilla and lower the heat to prevent burning.

Spoon the vegetable mixture on top. Add just enough shredded cheese to bind the ingredients. Allow to melt slightly, then add a few drops of hot sauce and spoon a small amount of salsa on top. Fold the tortilla. Turn the quesadilla over and heat on the other side for about a minute, then move to a plate and spoon salsa over it before serving.

That's a *perfect* day. They don't happen often. But they happen often enough that I lost the extra weight I'd gained back during relapse, plus more.

To look only at what I ate would be to miss the whole point of how I lost the weight. Despite behavioral and menu changes, one thing remains constant: I love food. It's one of the most sensual pleasures life has to offer. That attitude needn't change while you're losing or maintaining weight.

We didn't know back in Grandma's day what we know now about how to eat delicious food and still lose weight. One of the biggest laughs on the Internet is a site by writer Wendy McClure, who posted her collection of 1974 menu cards from Weight Watchers (http://www.candy boots.com/wwcards.html). There's nothing the least bit healthy, dietetic, or logical about these dreadful recipes; McClure calls them "unspeakably grim" and provides hilarious commentary, even savaging the props used in the photos: the Snappy Mackerel Casserole "is so snappy they've placed it in a special roped-off area!"

What greater (and more pointless) torture was there in 1974 than for an overweight person to dutifully whip up—using a heavy hand on the pimiento and dried onion flakes—such taste-tempters as Fluffy Mackerel Pudding, Chilled Celery Log, and Liver Pâté en Masque?

Today there's no excuse for hating your food while losing weight. But food cruelty abounds. Snack foods are sold to us in the guise of "real" food. As portions supersized over the years, savvy marketers convinced us that "energy" bars are health food, not candy bars; that bran muffins are reasonable breakfast choices, not dessert; that a Starbucks Frappuccino is a morning coffee drink, not a super-cal venti milkshake.

★ The Baked Apple of Her Eye

I ran into Sirius Radio host Lynn Samuels, she of the distinctive voice and opinions. Never shy about speaking her mind, Lynn assured me that *this* is what I should be eating for dessert:

Core an apple, sprinkle with cinnamon and a pinch of brown sugar, cook in microwave. How long should I cook it, Lynn? "Until it falls apart and melts on the plate."

Top with fat-free Reddi-wip. (Actually, you can top just about *anything* with fat-free Reddi-wip at 5 calories per serving.)

To appreciate food's pleasures, you have to make your portions appropriate. Desserts need to stay in their special place and not do a hostile takeover of the dinner plate. And low-quality, overprocessed, not-fresh, not-really-delicious food shouldn't be the mainstay of your diet; life's too short.

But not *so* short that you should use every opportunity to grab for the (tarnished) brass ring. "It's just this once," you reassure yourself as you OD on a special dessert.

Friends and well-wishers will be eager to hammer more nails in the coffin. "Relax, it's vacation! *It's just this once!*"

They'll say some variation of that on every vacation, weekend brunch, birthday and special occasion, dinner with friends, social event; really, anytime calories are within sight. You've had a long day! You've had a tough morning! You've never eaten in this particular restaurant with these particular friends before! You've never paired this appetizer with that wine! It's Thursday! Arbor Day comes only once a year—*enjoy!*

"Just this once" translates to "Just as always," and it's usually in the form of well-meaning pressure from someone who doesn't have to make the rounds with you as other food bullies take their place to ensure you're eligible for the sumo wrestler trainee program.

I recall a couple taking me out for my birthday where, after much consideration and inner struggle, I emerged clean, in control, and ready to face a new year by ordering (and looking forward to) the grilled vegetable platter. The woman squealed in horror, sounding genuinely angry: *You can't do that on your birthday!* It was as if I'd offered to tear the heads off baby chicks. I tried to explain that making this decision was difficult, something I'd long wanted to do, and that the decision, so recently birthed, was still tenuous and oxygen-deprived. It was a subject I'd spoken of to these friends many times, the hope that I would learn to feed myself healthfully rather than grabbing at what always seemed the final opportunity for something breaded and fried.

The woman and her husband went steely. There was no letup. They browbeat me, and in the face of such fury from my hosts, I caved. I ordered the chicken parmigiana, a favorite dish that accounts for a disproportionately large slice in the pie chart of my overall weight gain.

⭐ First Aid for Steamed Vegetables

Chef Terry sez: Steamed foods are boring by themselves, so I keep coulis in little squeeze bottles to dress them, liven them up, and decorate the edges of the plate. Coulis—from the Latin for "colander," or "to strain"—are basically puréed fruits or vegetables. They provide strong flavored accents that don't require much prep time or know-how. I make them potent because you don't need to use much. Coulis should be squiggled on the plate first; the food "floats" on top of it.

GINGER CARROT COULIS
(for fish, poultry, veggies)

4 large carrots, peeled and sliced thin
1 can chicken broth (water is okay,
*   but add 1 teaspoon salt)*
1 tablespoon powdered ginger

¼ teaspoon cayenne
Juice of 1 lime
1 garlic clove

Steam the carrots in the broth and add the ginger and cayenne. Add the lime juice and garlic. Cook until the carrots are soft, then allow to cool and purée in a blender.

ROASTED RED PEPPER COULIS
(No cooking here! Great with anything)

4 ounces roasted red peppers, drained
*   and rinsed*
3 garlic cloves (1 teaspoon garlic powder
*   okay)*
1 teaspoon basil (fresh basil leaves are best)

¼ teaspoon pepper
¼ cup olive oil
1 tablespoon balsamic vinegar

Combine and purée in a blender.

(continued)

COULIS TEX-MEX
(Great with anything)

3 ripe tomatoes, medium diced

1 small onion, medium diced

3 chopped garlic cloves

½ bunch scallions

1 tablespoon olive oil

½ teaspoon salt

Juice of 1 lime

½ teaspoon Tabasco

½ cup tomato juice or V8

½ teaspoon chili powder

Sauté the tomatoes, onion, garlic, and scallions in a fry pan with spray of olive oil until tender; set aside to cool. Place in a blender. Add the salt, lime juice, Tabasco, tomato juice (I use V8), and chili powder. Purée, then strain.

These people who bullied me are the unhealthiest eaters I know. Nominally vegetarians, they're contemptuous of salads or anything steamed, grilled, or otherwise nutritious. They eat only battered, deep-fried vegetables swimming in oils and creams. They're morally against gyms and anything requiring use of the body (*What are you, a machine?*), and have no concept of how the body is composed or functions. The woman hides her increasing tubbiness under voluminous men's shirts and artfully slung scarves. When I first began going to the gym and working out with a trainer, consequently trying to get to bed earlier than 3 A.M. so as to get a full night's rest, she reacted with alarm and bitterness at this betrayal of our friendship.

People who are wedded to unhealthy lifestyles are like devil worshippers who want you to chant alongside them in long black robes in the moonlight. *Come to the dark side! Stay up late and be a wreck tomorrow, like me!*

I'm no longer friendly with that couple. Ex-smokers stop hanging with smokers, the clean and sober stop mixing it up with druggies and drinkers, and people who get in shape begin to prefer the company of other healthy types. I'm not saying dump all your friends—just the ones who are food bullies. A solid, supportive friendship will weather your lifestyle changes. But you'd be surprised at how many friendships turn out to have been based on misery loving company. When I ordered that birthday vegetable platter, my companions betrayed genuine hostility because I wasn't in line with their antihealth mind-set. If I turned healthy, it would wipe out many of our social occasions (*let's eat till we're stupefied!*) and possibly put pressure on the couple to change as well. They both suffered from a range of mental and physical ailments, a few of which could have been ameliorated with exercise and proper nutrition, but instead they popped useless placebo pills from the "health food store." They worried about whether antibiotics or germs had gotten into their food supply, when it was their own chosen lifestyle that was poisoning them.

My sister can also be a food bully on occasion, even though she truly means well. We play a game called Drill Sergeant where she calls and asks how much progress I've made, then berates me into promising to do better. It's a game, but sometimes Diane brings unreasonable expectations to the table.

DIANE: "Are you going to eat healthfully today?"
ME: "Maybe."
DIANE: "'Maybe' isn't good enough!"
ME: [Muffled cursing]
DIANE: "Here's what you can have—a nice cold glass of water."

A nice cold glass of water? What kind of nutrition is that?

You can opt to cut off the real food bullies in your life (not my sister, of course). Unless the bully is the one who signs your paycheck. Consider the Borgata Babes, those serving wenches (and a few wench-men) of the Borgata casino in Atlantic City. They're suspended if they gain weight and sacked if they can't lose it again through company-mandated aerobics and nutrition classes. Pregnant employees—the casino has not yet taken steps to sterilize them—wear an expandable "transitional outfit" for 180 days before maternity leave.

Luckily for me, no one cares whether movie critics are fat; we're obscured in the shadows of screening rooms and come out of hiding like all journalists whenever there's an open bar. But you've got to keep those cocktail waitresses in line. A few extra pounds might make them lose their balance while serving drinks to men who are gambling away the family fortune (*I have a system!*), or perhaps the extra weight would pop the cross-straps of the Borgata's signature Zac Posen bustiers and endanger the guests. So it's a safety issue, really.

The Borgata casino is an extreme example of something that's pervasive in our society: food bullies who in some way hold the purse strings. It's not surprising that service-oriented businesses prefer to hire gorgeous (usually female) specimens. When the marketplace rules, only the young and beautiful—and slim—get hired. As a culture, we prefer slenderellas. But if the marketplace ruled, the overweight—that's 65 percent of America—would never get a job doing anything, anywhere. (Except as professional ballast or the occasional mob hit man.) Who'd be minding the store?

Every minority experiences subtle forms of oppression—in the workplace, when receiving medical care, while househunting. I'm not singling out fat people as the true sufferers in an uncaring world. (*You think the Holocaust was bad? Try being fat and ordering an ice cream sundae in public*

In the News: Deborah Voigt

When you're suicidal, what you need to wear is the perfect little black dress, and Deborah Voigt couldn't.

Voigt, who has been called "arguably the leading dramatic soprano singing today," was fired from a production of Strauss's *Ariadne auf Naxos* because she couldn't fit into the little black number that the director insisted was necessary for the role of the suicidally lovelorn Ariadne. Next we heard, Voigt had quietly undergone gastric bypass surgery and lost 100 pounds despite the risk of altering or damaging the quality of her voice.

Voigt claimed the surgery had *nothing to do* with that little black dress or a career threatened by fat-phobe directors.

and see the looks you get!) What fascinates me more than the Borgata hiring attractive people and using negative incentives to keep them that way (do it or you're fired) is the idea of the surprise weigh-in replacing the random drug test to keep employees in line. What strikes greater fear in a woman than reporting her actual weight?

Scale panic is pandemic in America. I can imagine women giving up their PINs to identity thieves sooner than they'd cop to where the scale was tipping. If you've ever witnessed a Weight Watchers weigh-in where women frantically divest themselves of stud earrings and run to take a last-minute pee to improve their chances, you can imagine the torment that accompanies the Borgata ritual, where there's something real at stake.

Fat as a consumable substance hasn't always been such an enemy. In 1977, about 45 percent of our calories came from fat, and while that was a powerful lot of fat, at least America was not yet a nation of elephants lumbering across the Disneyland veldt. That was the same year the national Dietary Guidelines for Americans made its first appearance—in the form of the famous Food Pyramid—to be revised every five years since. The most recent incarnation finally admitted that more fruit, vegetables, and whole grains are the way to go, and upped the exercise recommendations. (I still take exception to the design of the pyramid, because visually, the pinnacle represents the good stuff, the goal, and shouldn't be given over to the foods we're supposed to snub. How can you get excited about grains when they're on the dusty pyramid floor?)

MARIE'S LOW-FAT WINTER PASTA

This dish uses no fat in preparation, saving those calories for an optional cheese topping—or for an extra glass of wine with dinner. Marie calculated it at about eight "points," depending how much cheese you use.

SERVES 2

8 ounces broth (beef, chicken, or vegetable) or wine, or a combination
*   of broth and wine*
1 small white onion, coarsley chopped
3 garlic cloves
About ½ large bunch of broccoli
*About 8 to 10 sun-dried tomatoes reconstituted in water—*not *the ones*
*   packed in oil! (reserve water)*
4 ounces dried pasta or 8 ounces fresh pasta
Oregano, thyme, basil, red pepper flakes (varying amounts in that order)
Other vegetables to taste—zucchini, eggplant, red peppers—whatever looks
*   good in the market and would add texture*

A handful of flavorful mushrooms, such as shiitake, portobello, or hen-of-
the-woods
Salt and pepper to taste
2 to 3 ounces shredded or grated parmesan cheese or parmesan/romano mix

Boil the water for the pasta in a 3-quart pan.

Heat about half the broth in a high-sided sauté pan until it simmers. Add the onions and garlic and allow to soften. Add the broccoli and sun-dried tomatoes, since these take longest to cook. Reserve the liquid from the tomatoes to add later.

Add the pasta to the boiling water. Dried pasta takes about 10 to 12 minutes to cook; fresh pasta takes 4 to 6 minutes.

Add the herbs, red pepper flakes, and vegetables to the pan. As the cooking liquid evaporates, add the remaining broth, the liquid from the tomatoes, or a bit of wine (red for beef broth, white for chicken or vegetable). There should be a thin level of liquid (a bit more than ¼ inch deep) left in the pan when the vegetables finish cooking. Dense vegetables take longest to cook, so add the mushrooms last.

Use salt sparingly or not at all, since the broth and dried tomatoes contain salt.

When the vegetables are still slightly crunchy, drain the pasta and toss it with vegetable mixture over low-medium heat for about 2 minutes so the pasta can absorb some of the cooking liquid.

Top with fresh pepper and the cheese, and serve.

An alternative to grated hard cheese is a tablespoon of fresh ricotta or a large teaspoon of fresh goat cheese per serving; toss with the pasta to add a creamy texture.

The guidelines focused attention on how much fat we were consuming and helped turn the 1980s into a fat-free zone. Our ideal of feminine beauty became slimmer and more athletic; jogging was the newest craze, roller-skating was reclaimed from childhood, exercise became a religion. There was new interest in the health consequences of fat, including chronic disease and susceptibility to certain cancers. Between body consciousness and public health campaigns, America's fat intake decreased about 10 percentage points.

But that was within the context of a higher overall calorie intake. The general public thinks low-fat diets don't work because America happened to get fatter at the same time as the low-fat diet craze, when, in reality, everyone back then was eating a *high*-fat diet; *that's* why it didn't work. It's known as the SnackWells Syndrome because everyone thought "low-fat" on the packaging meant "eat the whole thing, it's good for you!" SnackWells cookies had less fat than similar-sized cookies of other brands, but after you eat 20 of them the benefit becomes moot.

The pendulum then swung to Atkins, a high-fat, no-carb diet in which you gorge yourself on bacon drippings. It's based on a kind of nutritional loophole in which, yes, technically you can lose weight by avoiding carbs. But the weight you're losing at first is mostly water, because that water is no longer needed to tend the glycogen stores. There's no more glycogen, a carb byproduct, to store. Later, also in the absence of carbs, the body literally eats itself from the inside out, gnawing on its own muscle and protein, in addition to fat.

Atkins devotees wind up on a restricted-calorie diet without realizing it. After the initial fun of marbled steak wears thin, Atkins followers get bored with eating heaps of protein and fat, and eventually feel unwell enough that they lose much of their appetite. You can lose weight this way, sure, but you pay a high price in terms of health. *And* you get bad breath.

⭐ Fiber Fact

Women who consume more whole grains weigh less than other women.

The Atkins fad let fat off the hook and recast carbs as the villain. It hurt sales of Krispy Kreme. It inspired thousands of new or retooled products, like "low-carb" ice cream that was *higher* in fat and calories than the original versions (and, from what I've sampled, pretty foul-tasting), yet was thought to be "healthy" because . . . aren't carbs the devil?

More than 3,000 low-carb products came on the market in 2004, according to industry groups. There was low-carb everything, even when it didn't make sense for that particular product. Low-carb peanut butter has the same number of calories as regular, so if you're eating more of it because you perceive it as "safer," it's the SnackWells Syndrome all over again, only with something that sticks to the roof of your mouth.

The tide has already turned on the low-carb craze. Modified plans like the South Beach Diet let you have *some* carbs in your life. You know Atkins is over when you hear that a hot new franchise is the California-based House of Bread.

But the SnackWells Syndrome lives on in every otherwise uplifting piece of nutritional news we get. People hear that olive oil is good for you, so they empty vats of it on their salads. Even foods that are genuinely healthful can be a sinkhole of calories and misery if you abuse them. The heroin addict plays Russian Roulette when he overdoses on his favorite substance, but people routinely abuse food day after day, fattening up for the slaughter, no trips to the ER (except for heart attacks and diabetic coma) to put a little perspective on how shabbily they're treating themselves.

Even if you're taking in a reasonable 25 percent fat in your overall diet, ask yourself this: 25 percent of *what*? Is it out of a daily dose of a million calories? Then all you're doing is the SnackWells Shuffle, sticking to the letter, not the spirit, of healthy eating.

★

I wanted to lose 100 pounds. I really believed I could. I probably still can.

But it's an unrealistic goal for now. By sticking rigidly to an arbitrary number, I was defying every precept I'd learned during my weight loss. It can't be about a number, it's got to be about specific changes in behavior and attitude.

After all, why did it have to be *100 pounds*? Because it sounded neat and dramatic. Because I said I would, and who're you calling a liar? Because I remember being 130 pounds in my early thirties and I wanted to have that body back, even though you can't go home again.

At HHHI, Bob Wright would trot out another of his famous phrases: Weight follows behavior. (Maybe not right away; JoAnne likes to say "it's in the pipeline.") No matter what grandiose plans you make or what number you pull out of your ass, your ideal weight is the one at which you're doing the most you're willing to do to keep it there. It's technically possible to get back to your high-school cheerleader weight, but the cost— eight hours a day in the gym and being seen in public with pom-poms— isn't worth it. No matter what you do and how you dare to dream, you'll wind up weighing a number on the scale you can live with, one that intersects at the precise point between what's mentally tolerable and what's physically sustainable.

So I changed my goal to 75 pounds. We'll see how that goes. Maybe down the road I'll attempt the last 25. You never know . . .

75 POUNDS:
HOLDING THE PUPPY

While I downsized my body, I was also scaling back other areas of my life that had run to excess—spending and accumulating. It was probably all linked to the same reason I got fat: emotional need. Why else did I accumulate so much *stuff* over the years?

When I moved, I had to go through all my *stuff* and decide how much of that *stuff* I wanted to take the time and effort to pack. Once you've packed 100 cartons of books and DVDs, you wonder how many more cartons you're going to need for all those papers and mementos and . . . *stuff*.

I began discarding. Helene from down the hall couldn't come home without finding another shopping bag of toys and videos for her kids hanging from her doorknob. Tim, a film professor upstairs, was the recipient of my laserdisc collection and player. I know laserdisc is the better medium, but I'm tired of saving full libraries of VHS, DVD, and LD the way I saved complete wardrobes of clothing in every size.

If there's ever a fire, I'll grab Tsuko, Buzz, and Sensei. Maybe some photo albums. That's all I need.

Not that I was prepared to get rid of everything except pets and photos; I wasn't planning on moving into a garret with only the clothes on my back.

Part of why I sold my apartment is that I suspected it was the height of the real-estate market and I wanted to cash out the equity I'd built up over nineteen years. I was also spurred in a strange way by my weight loss. It seemed I was ready to pare away excess and get back to basics in several facets of my life, beginning with my body, then spilling over into how and where I lived. I wanted more sunlight, for instance. I wanted access to trees and nature. I wanted to live somewhere less frenetic than my street in Chelsea, home to some of the hottest clubs I've never visited.

Plus, the new apartment had floor-to-ceiling windows and . . . you won't understand the thrill of this if you don't live in Manhattan, but it had a *washer/dryer* and a *kitchen-sink garbage disposal*! Be still my heart.

There was something more than market timing and amenities going on in my decision to move. Now that I was able to let go of clothing that didn't fit and fat that didn't suit me and papers and trinkets and *stuff*, the move was an acknowledgment that I was willing to let go of the past. For my streamlined new future, I wouldn't be needing a Xanadu, like the mansion Citizen Kane filled with detritus when all he really wanted was his Rosebud. It's not like my old place was so vast that I couldn't find my way to the East Wing, but it was actually larger than I needed, and the monthly maintenance was criminal.

Weight loss had everything to do with the move. Once you manage to change some of your ways, it's easier to look at the rest of your life and say, Hmmm, what needs fixing here? I could have lived the rest of my life in my gorgeous Chelsea Xanadu, with its planted terrace and 18-foot ceilings and Jacuzzi. One friend referred to it as the Pleasure Palace. But I was restless. Would I really live the rest of my life in the ground floor rear, no sunshine ever peeking through a window, and with a terrace ringed with barbed wire to keep burglars out?

I had the Xanadu and the *stuff*, the fancy Chelsea address and the hot clubs nearby with their limos blocking all the parking spaces. I've been fortunate to have these things, to have bought into Chelsea by blind luck when they were practically *giving* those apartments away.

Material things are lovely. But what's important is the Rosebuds. I miss my father; I know I can't have him back, but I can try to live in a way that would honor him. I worry about my mother now that she's entered her eighties and has pain from arthritis.

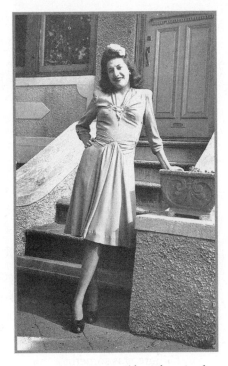

Mom at nineteen in Brooklyn. She never believed she was pretty!

We've always had a rocky relationship, my mother and I, probably because we're alike in so many ways. When I was in my twenties, she'd send me financial advice anonymously in envelopes with no return address—like blackmail notes, as if I didn't know who sent them! Did I heed her sensible advice to invest in money markets when the interest rates were double-digit? No! I saved nothing! Mom didn't know how to give and I didn't know how to accept. We have so many years to make up for now in such a limited amount of time.

I worry about my sister, Diane, who still zigs and zags through the stages of change without being able to commit to losing weight. "I think about it every day," she told me quietly in a taxi the other night as we were ferrying food to our mom.

For a highly verbal family, each of us desperate to do the Sunday

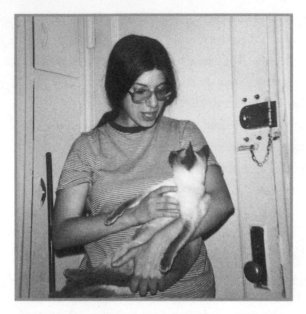

My sister, Diane, many years and pounds ago. With Seka.

crossword puzzle in ink, none of us could say those three little words. It was like trying to speak in that African "click" dialect. To this day, my sister won't let me hug her. Diary entry from December 27, 1964:

> *Today me and Diane tried to make cocoa ourselves. Diane put in vinegar and it tasted horrible. I wanted to cry in Diane's arms but she poked and pinched and punched real hard. I didn't cry but it hurt.*

One of the sweetest things Diane ever said was when I had breast cancer. I knew she was terrified, both for me and for herself. "Don't forget—you have a sister who loves you!" said Diane, my only sister.

The Rosebuds are important. The rest of the stuff, anything that can

164

be put in storage and then forgotten, doesn't need a big place in your life. Great books that I'll probably never read again don't need to stay on my shelf to remind me (or visitors) what good taste I have in literature. Childhood poems and cards and report cards are sweet; I saved the important ones and shredded the rest.

I got rid of what I didn't need—like my fat. I loved my fat, even though I claimed to hate it. Fat made me feel safe and protected. Perhaps that was an illusion, but fat felt necessary at the time.

And now it's not.

Weight loss isn't about numbers, it's about *change*. Most people find change terrifying and will do anything to avoid it. "Change bad!" I like to chortle, only half-kidding. The fear of change keeps people in abusive relationships or living uncomfortably with situations that could be improved with effort and courage. Often you don't know how unhappy you've been until you take a gamble on change and then experience a strange feeling—what is that, flu? Indigestion? No! It's *happiness*. It's contentment with yourself and your life and your body.

So *that's* what it feels like!

★

I became an early riser. It didn't happen overnight.

It's not just the zeal of the newly converted that goads me into saying that getting up early is better for you. I always suspected it despite a lifetime as a night owl. Studies indicate that people who work the lobster shift (that's what they call the midnight shift on newspapers) sleep fitfully and die younger; I don't doubt it. I worked the lobster shift a few times and never knew whether 6 A.M. was time for Wheaties or a rare steak.

My father was a night owl because of his job working the overnight mail trains, a now defunct holdover from the days of the Pony Express. (His job required him to carry a gun, which was . . . *thrilling*.) Whenever he had a day off, he slept through it. At night he'd come alive: snacking, watching detective movies on TV. I loved to join him. Staying Up Late With Daddy was cool.

In college, you naturally stay up all night so you can smoke pot, intone pretentious drivel about the universe, and feign maturity. Carly Simon sang, "I'm a night owl, honey" in a sexy growl that implied life was more interesting in the wee hours.

When I began working at the *New York Post* while I was still in college, I was on the swing shift, which ended at 1 A.M.—just in time for carousing at bars in the Village with seasoned, grizzled reporters who bought me drinks in return for my listening wide-eyed to their stories of reportorial derring-do. Then we'd go to after-hours joints serving liquor illegally and we'd dance and drink and stumble out into the grayish morning light.

Even after I'd tired of the endless loop of stories from the old-timers about back in the day, I continued to stay up late. Bedtime was 3 A.M. I justified it every which way. I'm a *creative artist,* we don't get up early in the morning! This was how Daddy lived! I'm wild, dangerous . . . a night owl, honey!

Mornings were late, bleary-eyed, slow to get revved.

Bad sleeping habits provide a trail of crumbs that leads right to . . . carbs, that interplay of hormones and hunger triggers that comes unglued with lack of sleep.

This is an example of how, to lose serious weight, you've got to examine cherished ideals about yourself. Was I really a night owl? Did I have to stay that way?

To increase your chances you've got to create a living environment that makes weight loss not only attractive but inevitable. For that, you might have to let go of ancient, stubborn views of yourself and all the rationalizations you built in support of those views: *If I go to bed an hour earlier, I'll be giving up my individuality and my constitutionally protected right to stay up all night and wreck my health!*

Not to sound too Zen, but I didn't give up anything I wasn't ready (and happy) to part with. I'd been in love with the romance of the idea of staying up late. I'd ignored how bad it made me feel in the morning, how out of step I was with friends and services and possibilities. And the sunrise.

I'd love to tell you I purposely changed my sleep patterns to capitalize on the health benefits of a good night's rest. But I did it begrudgingly, and mainly because the 7 A.M. body-sculpt class was the only time Diane Stefani could make it to the gym with me. I needed a gym buddy, a minder, more than sleep.

I dragged myself out of bed to meet her, cursing all the way. Diane is a sweetheart and I didn't want to let her down, but being a dependable and responsible friend turns out to be just as much work as losing 75 pounds. I lived a mere half block from the gym, yet rarely made it on time for the warm-up. Diane was always there reading the papers before the class started, despite having to schlep in from Queens laden with a change of clothes on hangers plus all manner of wheeled luggage.

There are books that explain step by step how to reset your body clock, how to get up 10 minutes earlier every day, how to fool and reframe your biology. It requires an Einstein's worth of mathematical calculations; let's see, what time does the sun rise in this latitude?

I didn't do it like that. I sullenly slammed the alarm clock off each morning, changing neither habit nor attitude, grimly determined to make it to a few gym classes a week. But secretly, magically, like little elves finishing the cobbler's shoes during the night, my body and brain chemistry reset themselves. After a year of this, the unthinkable happened: I now wake up every morning sans alarm by 6:30. Sometimes earlier. And in a fairly decent mood. I try to whisper to myself, "It's Saturday! Go back to sleep!" But I prefer to jump up and get started on the day. I've got *spilkes*.

I've become the type of person I used to deride as too dull: Normal. In step. A nice girl from Queens.

★

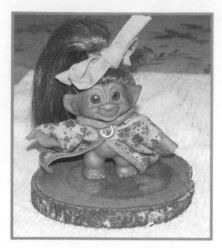

The purloined Troll doll.

One summer in the Poconos when Susan and Sharon in the bungalow next door got a new puppy, they threw a party.

"Who wants to hold the puppy?" asked their mom.

All the kids clamored for it, but I must've looked the most desperate—Baby Dear the hamster was the highest up the pet chain Diane and I seemed likely to climb at the time—so I promptly sat on the throne of a hardwood kitchen chair with a sleepy, furry ball of bewildered puppy in my arms. This was way better than stroking the purple-haired Troll doll I'd swiped from Susan and Sharon the summer before.

(No, I've never stolen money, but I took the Troll doll and also liberated a few memo pads from McCrory's 5&10.)

Then it all began to go wrong. I proudly held the puppy as the other kids lined up for cake and soda. Everyone was served except me. "Can I have some too?" I asked, Oliver-style, throat constricted. I was struggling with the same anxiety I'd experienced when all the ice creams had been handed out at day camp and I hadn't gotten one.

Susan and Sharon's mother was stern. "You're holding the puppy," she said, as if I could see the apparent logic in this.

It was a crushing blow. I wouldn't have volunteered for puppy patrol had I known there were conditions. And yet it was as if I'd been given a special honor, a responsibility for which not every nine-year-old was qualified. I had an assignment, a mandate, a mission.

That afternoon, I got to hold the puppy *and* I had my cake and ate it too—although delayed gratification sucks. Children have it right when they kick and scream on the floor if they don't get what they want *now*.

In weight loss, as in life, you trade something nice now for something better later on. While I was losing the 75 pounds, I sometimes resented that in some larger sense, everyone was having cake and ice cream without me. I'd have to ground myself in the immediacy of my weight-loss goals—aesthetic, healthwise, and more—until I could turn off the Pavlovian salivary faucets and remember:

Maybe someday. Right now, I'm holding the puppy. And that is reward enough.

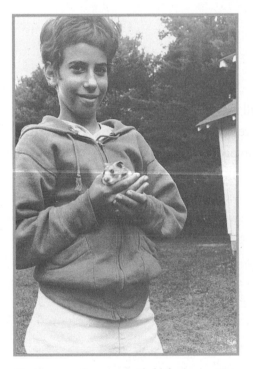

The Poconos, the summer I held the puppy. Here I am holding Baby Dear the hamster. Mom sent us to the nearby beautician trainee school where they gave you free haircuts if you let the students practice on you; you get what you pay for. *(Photo by Sam Bernard)*

Part Two

★

THE KNACK, AND HOW TO GET IT

READY . . . OR NOT

Losing weight is like that "daughter-sister" line in "Chinatown": It's hard. It's easy. It's hard. It's easy.

It's hard *and* it's easy.

If there weren't so many emotional issues tied to weight gain, or so many subterranean biological currents, losing weight would be a snap. You've no doubt done it yourself—started a diet, lost weight, then scrapped the diet, only to see the pounds return like those boomerang kids who come home to Mommy after their midlife breakdowns. "Didja keep my room the way I left it?"

You want to lose weight. But you don't want to, for unfathomable reasons. You want to *and* you don't.

Before I resolved to lose 100 pounds (which turned into 75), I knew there were still emotional issues in play. I decided, Screw it, I'll just lose the weight and face those issues as they pop up.

Pop up they did. I had a backlog worthy of Family Court with so many personal issues on the docket. As I considered each issue, I didn't always like what they said about me. True, I'm not a murderer. I don't kite checks, hold up small convenience stores, bully children, or plot the downfall of governments. Still, the truth can hurt. Once I opened the floodgates to self-knowledge, a rush of sludge poured in: Bad behavior! Foot-in-mouth disease! Schadenfreude!

★ Sobering Thought for the Day

Your body has between 30 billion and 40 billion fat cells.

I was willing to tackle these issues, though. Sometimes it's simply the willingness to be honest with yourself that gives you the confidence to behave better next time around.

Once you move all that emotional baggage to a different luggage carousel, one where someone else will probably steal it, losing weight becomes relatively easy. You just need to know how: information, technique, and especially practice. It definitely gets easier with practice.

In the following chapters, I'll give you a preview of how to lose weight on your own should you decide to go that route. This is just a taste of the possibilities, not a prescription. But remember, no matter how bossy and self-righteous I can sound (I'm working on that, okay?), I'm not a health professional, a $1,000-an-hour behaviorist, or a golf-playin', cold-stethoscope-lovin' physician. Any weight-loss program must begin with a visit to the doctor to check for underlying medical conditions. I don't want this book recalled like one of those malfunctioning heart-valve devices: *Gee, I read Jami's book and suddenly I keeled over!* If I say "exercise till you drop," for example, I'm using HUMOR, and you should skip that advice and move on to something less controversial, like "eat rutabaga."

But first, here's the big question: Do you really want to lose weight?

I know, I know. You'd give your right arm to lose a few pounds.

Good news: You won't have to give up any limbs! Neither will you have to renounce your favorite foods, starve yourself, or suffer the flames of hell.

⭐ The Naked Woman

We're *supposed* to be fat. What a relief.

In *The Naked Woman: A Study of the Female Body*, by zoologist Desmond Morris—and yes, I'm a little insulted that it took a *zoologist* to reach this conclusion—we learn all about the wonders of neoteny, the presence of rounded features that instills in mothers the patience not to throttle their babies (*Ooh, he's so cute when he screams!*) and in men the urge to protect women. Our "childlike, rounded features" are "attractive and endearing."

That doesn't mean you can push back in the La-Z-Boy and pop open another brewski. If you've been going around boasting you'd give your right arm to lose weight at the same time as swearing you'll never give up deep-fried Mars bars, then you're just not ready.

In Chapter 2, I discussed the "click," that moment when losing weight makes sense and feels nearly effortless. It happens at a certain point along the "stages of change," a five-part continuum of behaviors and attitudes typical of those trying to kick addictions—in this case, an addiction to abusing food.

First, is it possible to "abuse" food?

Are you kidding me with that question? Overeating might not be the stuff of literary and medical drama the way drug abuse is, but the behavior is no different—addictive, self-destructive. Go to any weight-loss spa and listen to the newbies whine and moan because they're going "cold turkey" on 1200 calories a day. It's not the food they're addicted to—we all have to eat—it's the behavior. Hot-dog-eating contests? *Food abuse!* Thanksgiving every day? *Food abuse!*

There are people who say, Relax. It will happen when you're ready. But it doesn't just "happen," you've got to *make* it happen by taking action. At the same time, you probably won't make a serious effort until you're in an appropriately receptive frame of mind. To get a fix on where you stand, how receptive you really are to change, try to locate yourself along the stages of change:

Pre-contemplation

This is where you probably don't think you have a problem, or if you do, you have no intention of fixing it. If someone politely suggests you stop pouring sugar down your throat through a funnel, and your response is to pull out your granddaddy's shotgun and lock and load for bear, then you're still in pre-contemplation. We'll just tiptoe away now and leave you be.

Coaxing someone out of pre-contemplation is tricky. People stuck here don't respond well to threats, preaching, or tough love. They shrug at morbidity and mortality statistics; if you wag a finger, they bite it off (and ask for seconds).

I was in pre-contemplation for years. I wanted to do something about that pesky little weight problem, I really did—but wait, wasn't it time to clean the computer keyboard with alcohol and a Q-tip, one key at a time?

One of my favorite readers, Irwin, had gotten up to 535 pounds before his doctor threatened to start writing his eulogy. It wasn't the amorphous prospect of death that moved Irwin to lose weight but something more tangible. "I had a young child at home who was about to lose her father. Today, twenty-eight years later, I weigh about 233. Not only have I lost more than 300 pounds, but I have kept the majority of the weight off for over twenty-five years. My daughter recently presented me with a grand-daughter."

If you're dimly aware that you haven't let anyone take your picture in ten years, and you think an entire box of doughnuts is a "suggested serving," then rest assured you're still in pre-contemplation. Keep a syringe of insulin handy.

Contemplation

The transition to this stage probably won't occur until you strip away all rationalizations and see yourself as you really are.

Which is to say, fat. Not pleasingly plump, or round, curvy, stout, or zaftig, but *fat*.

"I have a glandular problem" and "I just like food a lot" are the kinds of things you say when you're in pre-contemplation. When you add, ". . . and food makes me feel safe and in control," you're ready to graduate to contemplation, where you're open to possibilities, even if the idea of acting on them brings on an emergency nap. It's a dangerous time because nothing says you *can't* take an emergency nap or that you *have* to advance in life. No behavior cops will ticket you for loitering: "Move along, miss, you're scaring the children!"

Preparation

This is where the rubber starts to meet the road—you make bona fide plans to take action.

For most of her adult life, my sister has ducked her head out of contemplation and right back in, like Punxsutawney Phil forecasting the next six weeks of winter. Occasionally she'll venture out of her burrow briefly to visit the preparation stage. Diane takes perverse pride in never having exercised in her life, but she joined a gym one day while wafting along on a stray, gossamer strand of stage three preparation fever. She bought the necessary workout clothes and footwear and took an introductory weight-training session. It left her aglow with excitement and her very first endorphin rush, which she greeted like a child her first snowfall.

"I feel great! This is *amazing!*" she said.

"That's the endorphins."

"I can't believe it! I want to do my laundry and change the old shower curtain! What *is* this stuff?"

"It's the *endorphins.*"

She never went back.

For reasons unknown, or no reason at all, Diane fled back to the safety of the burrow of contemplation. Six more weeks of winter! Six more years of sloth!

It doesn't invalidate the start she tried to make. The more times she ventures into preparation, the easier it will be to stay there. At least now she's got the clothes.

During the preparation stage, I acted as if I were going for a Ph.D. in nutrition. I read all the literature; I subscribed to health newsletters from trusted sources like Tufts and the Mayo Clinic. I studied photos in Arnold Schwarzenegger's *Encyclopedia of Modern Bodybuilding* to learn about the muscle groups, what they do, and where they attach, so I'd be ready for the day some gym instructor named Bambi might squeal, *"Work those lats!"*

In the preparation stage, you might even pick up a dumbbell. You'll probably set it right down again, but at least you're laying the groundwork for weight loss by positioning yourself where it's more likely to happen. After all, joining a gym brings you that much closer to the treadmill.

When you actually step on that treadmill, you've entered the next stage.

Action

Here you physically, demonstrably modify your behavior in order to meet your goals. Perhaps you go on a diet, cook meals to prepackage for the week ahead, count calories. Whatever you're doing, it's visible, no longer in the realm of fantasy. You're out there creating new habits, scything your way through the underbrush. The audience is going wild.

That weight-loss epiphany that everyone reports occurs during the synapse between preparation and action, when you're pushing through the ether from "I plan to do something" to "I'm doing something."

Click!

This is the moment of clarity and exhilaration. As you stand balanced on the border between stages three and four, all is possible. The world is your oyster—and oysters, if they're not deep-fried and you don't have a shellfish allergy, are only 70 calories for three ounces of the Pacific kind, raw.

Everything you did during the preparation stage was part of getting to the action stage. Overcoming an addiction to overeating isn't measured on the scale, it's measured in the progress you make along these stages of change. So even when you move back and forth between stages (a normal and expected part of the process), you're still working on the problem, the machinery clanking in the background.

You haven't "blown it" when you temporarily retreat from the action phase. Successful weight losers make about seven stabs at it before they're successful.

Don't get me wrong—I'm in thrall to the bathroom scale. I hop on it nearly every day, sometimes more, like a smoker sneaking cigarettes. I've crowed over the tiniest loss and gone barking mad when the needle moved in the wrong direction. I've even placed the scale on the precise bathroom tile that gives the least weighty bang for the buck.

But the scale measures only one type of success—not inches lost, muscle gained, or lessons learned.

It's possible to lose some weight during the preparation stage, but in the action stage, your fat cells wail like the Wicked Witch of the West: "I'm melting!"

But it's not over. There's one stage left, and if you skip it, you're dead meat, the well-marbled kind.

Maintenance

Unglamorous, unsexy. The admiring crowds have packed up and gone home. But it's in maintenance that you do the work of ensuring weight-loss success.

Gird your loins—maintenance includes setbacks. Possibly relapses. I regained 10 pounds during my weight-loss journey and had to fight them off again. Setbacks are a necessary and integral part of the whole she-bang; it's the very act of overcoming them, time and again, getting more proficient at it with each success, that solidifies your overall achievement. As Bob Wright from HHHI says, "This is where you are more of the new behavior than the old behavior. There's a debate in your head, but you're leaning in the new direction."

What to do if you backslide, if you lose the "click" and feel stuck again? You need to push yourself ahead to the perimeter of preparation and again poise yourself to leap. You can do that by acting as if you're already there, imitating the behaviors and attitudes you might have in the stage you're aiming for even when your heart's not in it.

The preparation stage is necessary and helpful. But you can drum your fingers in it for an eternity. To force the bloom, even if you don't feel like it or don't believe this will work, you need to do something active, to imitate a behavior that belongs to the action stage of change:

Eat one healthy meal.

Take one vigorous walk.

Do one active thing.

Compound that with other tools at your disposal: behavior modification; keeping a food diary; shopping the perimeter of a supermarket, where you're more likely to find fruits, vegetables, and healthful items.

Force yourself to do one or more of these things, even if you believe you have no intention of keeping at it. The click will click into place sooner than you think. The more times you move from stage three to stage four, the sooner it clicks. Practice is such a strong conditioner that veteran bulimics don't even put a finger down their throats; they can upchuck at will.

Don't stop short of getting to—and through—maintenance. This is precisely where people tend to go off the rails. They see the nice number on the scale, and they take their bows and a premature victory lap. But if you don't work just as hard to move into the fifth stage of change, you can slide all the way down the slope to the lumpen land of pre-contemplation.

Enjoy the chips and dip.

WHO'S YOUR DADDY?

You want weight-loss advice? There's no shortage of it.

In 1898, businessman Horace Fletcher dropped 40 pounds by chewing his food until it turned to liquid; "Fletcherism" became all the rage.

In 1905, the La Grecque Corset was so tight it was thought to flatten the tummy permanently.

In 1910, Phytoline tablets were in vogue. Ingredients included arsenic and strychnine.

William the Conqueror made history. Forget about the Battle of Hastings and how he created the first census; he invented the liquid diet in 1087. The liquid: alcohol.

More liquid diets: In the 1600s, George Cheyne got milk, and *only* milk. In 1811, Lord Byron poured vinegar on his food and lost 64 pounds, if not a star in Ye Olde Michelin Guide.

Some of history's diet gurus invented their own foods: There's James

Salisbury and the Salisbury steak (take with hot water), the Reverend Sylvester Graham and the Graham cracker (take with water and vegetables), and the cereal maker and avowed Fletcherite John Harvey Kellogg and his granola (I presume he wanted it taken with milk or while wearing Birkenstocks).

Today we've got ever more liquid fasts, plus "energy" bars and "supplements"—like the subsequently banned heart-stopper fen-phen.

And we've got pundits. Lots of pundits. Americans spend $42 billion a year on diet and health books; simply lugging them home from Barnes & Noble is a weight-bearing exercise.

In the phenomenally annoying book *French Women Don't Get Fat*, Mireille Guiliano congratulates herself on being culturally attuned to slenderness as if it's her birthright. Or since she sprinkles her book with French words to fulfill the requirements of her publishing niche, slenderness must be her *drôit de naissance* (which is not an actual French expression but sounds as legitimate as some of Guiliano's theories).

The only thing that ever spoiled this woman's bliss was a trip to America when she was a teenager. She promptly gained 20 pounds from all that bad influence *Américain*. Forced to eat calorie-dense bagels standing up—something like that—she then hauled her newly fat *derrière* back to *La France*, where there's a civilized respect for food and the body, only to have her father greet her by comparing her to a sack of *pommes de terres*.

The way she tells it, she had a session with someone she calls "Dr. Miracle," who told her to stop eating pastries. Surely you don't have to pay a doctor—either French, miraculous, or *je ne sais quois*—to tell you *that*.

Because she is able to keep her girlish figure to this day, even though she eats multicourse meals in restaurants 300 times per *année* as part of her work as a CEO of Veuve Clicquot, Guiliano draws the conclusion that French women are naturally thin, that they have a healthy relationship with food, that they don't obsess over kilos, and that moderation comes as naturally to them as a *canard* to *l'eau*. (She likes *canard*, or duck, but claims that the French don't give a damn about *dinde,* or turkey, which is lower in fat and calories.)

I love the French. I love their food, language, culture. So what if they hate us? But give me a break—not all French women are thin, and that's for starters. You see slender women on St.-Germain de Prés just as you do on Madison Avenue because Paris and New York are cities with a major confluence of wealth and style. If you go out in the countryside to a festival *du fromage,* you'll probably see where they've been hiding all the French women who *do* get fat.

Obesity is a growing problem in France as in other developed countries. Do they not have a McDonald's on the Champs-Elysées? There are at least seven European countries that are officially fatter than America; France is not among them, but obesity in *les femmes* rose from 8 percent in 1997 to 11.3 percent in 2003, with slightly higher statistics for *les hommes.*

Guiliano is right to advocate a sensible approach to savoring fine food. Yet she starts off her Gallic eating plan with 48 hours of leek soup, which sounds just as wacky and obsessive as those omnipresent detox regimens rooted in fear and loathing of the body. Where is the nurturing and sensible eating in 48 hours of leek soup?

"While your leeks are boiling"—oh, yum—she advises you to ask yourself why you want to lose weight. "[Is it] because I'm afraid my husband or girlfriends think I am *bouboum* (overweight and dumpy)?"

One op-ed writer observed that the real reason so many Parisian women are slim is that they chain-smoke. So healthy, zee French.

I'm not inclined to take diet advice from a woman whose sole credentials on the topic are that she once gained 20 pounds, when she was nineteen. Who doesn't gain 20 pounds at that age? The Freshman 10, the Freshman 20, it's a cherished rite of passage that usually coincides with a teenager's first time away from parental control and supervised meals. When I got to college I weighed 117 pounds, yet was under the impression that cheesecake was a smart breakfast choice. My roommates were amused, possibly frightened, but no one thought to sign me up for Nutrition 101. The morning cheesecake continued unabated.

A 20-pound gain at that age could be nothing, just a case of advanced baby fat. So I don't want some lightweight *bouboum* telling me, "Hey, I have a nice body and I make my own yogurt, so that must be the key to success!"

In the News: "Real" Women

In what is either a breakthrough in the depiction of women or just a savvy marketing fad, Dove began using hefty, nonmodel models in their ads under the banner "Campaign for Real Beauty"—"because real beauty comes in many shapes, sizes and ages." But the ads are hawking "Intensive Firming Cream" so that these "real" beauties can anxiously try to get rid of their cellulite.

Other companies are hopping on the "real women" bandwagon. A Nike ad that reads like something from Maya Angelou's reject pile goes,

My butt is big
And round like the letter C. . . .
To those that walk behind me
It's a border collie
That herds skinny women
Away from the best deals
At clothing sales.

Today, everyone's got a diet for you. Whom can you trust?
For starters, you can rule out celebrity diets. "The Hotel Chain

Heiress' Guide to Staying Trim Through Promiscuous Sex" book is no doubt useful to hotel heiresses. That doesn't mean her words of wisdom would be right for *you.*

It's natural to look to celebrities for style tips. Would the eighties have even existed without Meg Ryan's haircut? But turning celebs into nutritional role models is dicey. Renée Zellweger presents the awesome spectacle of deliberately putting on 20 pounds—twice!—for the *Bridget Jones's Diary* movies, then slimming down again to stick-figure proportions. She reportedly received an extra $225,000 for every kilo of weight she added, and that was on top of her $15 million salary. If we were in a primitive culture but with a modern sense of body anxiety, Zellweger would be worshipped as a shape-shifting goddess.

It's quite a feat, gaining and losing on contract. But one that's not without a price. However Zellweger chose to lose the weight afterward, she seems to have gone too far, losing along with it some of the appealing roundness she displayed in the first *Bridget Jones.* She provides a binge/purge behavioral model even if she never binged or purged.

There are fat actresses I admire for being quintessentially themselves: Kathy Bates, Camryn Manheim, to name two. Kate Winslet is hardly fat, but she's unapologetically *womanly.* Some supermarket tabloids complained Winslet was in danger of being buried in a piano case when she dared balloon to a size 14 once, but Winslet then and now, and no doubt forever, looks fantastic and, more important, seems comfortable in her skin.

In Manheim's amusing memoir *Wake Up, I'm Fat!,* she describes becoming an activist in the increasingly militant movement for fat acceptance, where people embrace their large bodies instead of trying to change them.

I love how Manheim accepted her 1998 Emmy for *The Practice* with a shout-out: "This is for all the fat girls!" In the abstract, the idea of loving your body is a wonderful thing. Still, I have doubts about the Fat Power movement. It smacks of the Stockholm Syndrome, where people in captivity begin to side with their kidnappers: *Yeah, I'm a prisoner of my fat, but it feeds me five squares a day!*

It's certainly better to love your body than not. And it's important not to buy into cultural preconceptions of what a body should look like. But the problem here is the same that I have with the unconditional self-acceptance movement: Are we congratulating ourselves with reason? For actual accomplishment? For things to be proud of? Or are we just patting ourselves on the back for the sake of it out of some misplaced democratizing instinct in which we refuse to pass judgment on anyone or anything?

In some ways, the case for American obesity has been overstated. Figures were fudged. (Fudge? I just looked up like a prairie dog!)

Nevertheless, fat is more than an annoyance. Over time, fat people tend to get fatter unless there's an intervention. Overweight is a hindrance in the job market and a predictor of serious health problems. Yes, love your body, by all means! But don't love your fat to the degree where you convince yourself you're off the hook about staying healthy.

In my mid-thirties, I protested that the national argument over fat didn't really hinge on "health" but on culturally defined aesthetics and prejudices. I spoke in ignorance, not knowing what it might feel like to grow old with fat, to succumb to Type 2 diabetes, knee problems, sleep apnea, stroke, you name it. I assumed that because I felt fine, it would always be thus.

Today, the connection between cigarettes and lung cancer is unmistakable. Canadian cigarettes carry full-color photos of mouth and lung cancers. But the diffuse connection between fat and the long list of ailments it can exacerbate is harder to grasp, and I doubt there'll come a day when Christmas-cookie tins carry photos of coronary patients.

If you're fat, you have two basic options: you can hate it or embrace it.

Most people move uneasily between those options, too ambivalent to commit either way.

Even among the African-American community, where it's assumed that larger bodies remain acceptable and appealing, clinics have noted a rise in eating disorders among young girls. Beneath the bravado of any fat-acceptance movement is the harsh reality of what people really believe or how they act in private. Better self-esteem isn't the sole cure for the tangle of issues and emotions that characterize body dysmorphia, a disease mostly affecting women who are severely conflicted about their appearance.

The most famous "fat actress," Kirstie Alley, troubles me. I'm no carnival barker who can size up anyone's weight to the ounce, but Alley daintily claimed on *Oprah* that her peak was 219 pounds. *That's 219 pounds in one butt cheek, lady!* Why be coy?

I don't mean to denigrate a sister-in-dimpled-arms, but the self-proclaimed "fat actress" had, at the time of her cable-TV series, the biggest ass I've ever seen. Even Oprah proclaimed it a "sistah-butt." Alley later lost weight in her well-publicized role as spokesfatperson for Jenny Craig, but when she made *Fat Actress*—a ballsy and profitable move—her ass was the biggest thing in showbiz.

She was still gorgeous. Still funny. A big ass doesn't diminish a person's worth, despite jokes (and fears) to the contrary. I just wish she'd gone the extra mile and owned up to her real weight in all its fleshy majesty.

Alley's reality-esque TV series lampooned her real-life situation: a stunner whose weight cost her job opportunities, whose amplitude was distorted by unbecoming paparazzi shots.

In the first episode, Alley—playing a peekaboo version of herself—buries her misfortunes in a fast-food wallow in her car. The series flirted with the ever-expanding boundaries of Alley's panty line and how far you can push the limits of fat discourse in a fat-phobic industry. The show was daring, though not brilliant—perhaps because Alley's vanity was still weirdly attached. She was willing to make herself the butt of jokes, as she often did on *Cheers*, but she wasn't ready for a full-body immersion in her discomfort zone. *Fat Actress* needed to be unapologetically *fat* to extend itself the full length of the creative limb.

Alley didn't want to defy her critics, she wanted what they wanted—to return to her old, slim self. This desire bled through in the interviews she gave, percolating down to the essence of the show itself. The humiliation of fat could be done for laughs, the fat-phobes in Hollywood exposed—but on some level, Alley hungered to be on the other side of the looking glass. She used *Fat Actress* as a calling card to cash in on her career dilemma; to remind everyone of her talent; to secure the Jenny Craig deal; and then to run like hell from the sexy gal with the fat ass.

In one episode, her character tries to lose weight on a diet with a "think small" philosophy that has her hanging with little people. In another, her real-life friend and neighbor John Travolta stops by; Travolta's revolted. Alley has said that Travolta really did give her lectures on her need to lose weight. The squirm factor for me wasn't the tease between comedy and reality, or between the safe and the politically incorrect. It was that, fundamentally, the show was dishonest; Alley wasn't siding with her protagonist.

The show was a breakthrough of sorts—certainly better than *The Biggest Loser*, the reality-based series that humiliated competitive teams of fatties, but left a greasy aftertaste. Alley used it as a candied carrot on a stick to get the Jenny Craig endorsement deal. (She admitted as much on *Oprah*, that *she* went after *them*.) I can't fault her for pursuing a high-stakes, big-bucks opportunity. What I hate is the calculated synergy combined with what appears to be a relentless self-loathing.

On the November 7, 2005, *Oprah*, Alley said her "before" pictures made her "want to throw up." I'm not crazy about my "before" pictures either. When I look at them, I roll my eyes. They make me feel sad because it's painful to be fat and because I now see I've had so many bad haircuts over the years.

But although I hated being fat, I didn't hate *myself*. This is a distinction that gets lost when Alley carelessly promotes Jenny Craig as an antidote for wanting to throw up when you look at yourself. As a spokesfatperson, Alley is in a delicate position most of us will never face, where she can influence how others feel about their bodies, hence how they spend their money on "remedies." So when Alley sides in public with those who are disgusted by fat, that's when Camryn Manheim should burst in on her motorcycle with a gang of her fat-proud friends and knock Alley off Oprah's high-visibility couch.

Clearly Alley lost a chunk of weight, Photoshop notwithstanding, and made a chunk of change. On *Oprah,* where she looked terrific (while far from svelte), she claimed the total was 55 pounds, 40 to go.

Personally, I don't care if Alley is fat or thin. I love her (usually). She's funny. And that amazing shimmer in her amazingly luxuriant hair! What I mind is that she disingenuously fudges the numbers while profiting from them, like giving a stock tip in which she has a vested interest.

In truth, she's turned her back on herself—and, by extension, on all of us—by disavowing her former fat-actress self. Alley will never give a Manheim cheer to "all the fat girls." In a newspaper column after episodes of her show were rushed to DVD as if they were the director's cut of *Citizen Kane,* she said, "I'd always said it doesn't matter if I'm fat. But now that I'm not fat, I'm like, eww."

Eww? Is she talking about *us?*

Okay, can't trust celebrities. What else can't we trust?

Chuck any diet that tries to sell you special vitamins, supplements, or formulations along with it. That's not a diet, it's a sales pitch. Follow the first rule of consumer protection: Be wary of information— on nutrition, stocks, shares in uranium mines—from people who have a financial interest in it. "You'll lose weight if you buy this thing from me for $100" should raise your eyebrow, not quicken your pulse.

Ignore diets that promise quick, dramatic weight loss or that demonize entire food groups. There was a "fat blocker" a few years back (the Federal Trade Commission was all over it) that promised, "Blast up to 49 pounds off you in only 29 days!"

Skip over claims to share nutritional secrets the government is suppressing. The government can barely build a levee, let alone keep a burning secret about supplements or drugs that allow you to lose weight, cure cancer, *and* do windows. There are certainly some drugs out there that make you lose weight—you can score them in the darkest alleys on the edge of town. Prescription drugs that help you lose weight are another thing, but again, use cautiously and only under a doctor's care—so far, they all have nasty side effects or other downsides you might not want to risk.

Don't go crazy with herbal diet teas that promise results. People have died from overusing the laxatives and diuretics to be found in them, and in lower doses they can cause cramps, nausea, electrolyte imbalance, and fainting. It's just another example of how there is no substitute, or supplement, for the health benefits of a balanced diet. My guess is you are *not* suffering from a depletion of one micro-mineral that can't be found in your regular one-a-day multivitamin.

I'm so good at ferreting out quackery I can tell when a book or website is not to be trusted *simply by the typeface.* I'm not kidding! Quacks seem to be drawn by unseen forces toward choosing ugly, fussy, confidence-killing typefaces!

★ Calorie Alert

A Barbacoa Burrito with all the trimmings at Chipotle is 1270 calories. Healthier alternative: the Chicken Burrito Bol (without cheese, rice, or guacamole), 430 calories.

Be suspicious of extreme ways of eating, especially when they're for the dubious purpose of ridding the body of "toxins." Exactly what toxins are these? They're never specified. They're talked about in hushed tones, as in "There are toxins in my body and someone is wiretapping my brain!"

Don't use nouns as verbs. Okay, I know that advice belongs in a book on grammar like *Eats, Shoots, & Leaves.* But please don't say "juicing" around me. Why ruin a perfectly nice noun? If you love fresh juice, fine. If you drink only juice (and a little potassium broth) for that light-headed, euphoric feeling you get from fasting, also fine—even if you mistake it for higher consciousness or religious revelation.

But don't "juice" on the presumption it will cleanse your body of "toxins." It reminds me of how they convinced women in the 1950s to douche (which is actually harmful) on the seemingly sensible idea that vaginas need a spring cleaning. It's all just hype and body fear (if not downright misogyny). As Stephen Barrett, vice president of the National Council Against Health Fraud, points out on his essential (and highly entertaining) website Quackwatch (www.quackwatch.org), "The enzymes in plants help regulate the metabolic function of plants. When ingested, they do not act as enzymes within the human body, because they are digested rather than absorbed intact into the body. . . . And sensible eating, which is not difficult to do, furnishes an adequate nutrient supply."

Beware of diets with stupid names. Remember the "diet candy" plan with the unfortunate title "Ayds"? The FTC cracked down on it in 1944 for claiming it could help you "lose up to 10 pounds in 5 days, without dieting or exercising." The law didn't crush them, but in the early eighties, an acronym did.

An exception to the stupid-name rule might be Volumetrics, which encourages eating large quantities of food by choosing the ones that take up more space on your plate and in your stomach. Although the title sounds like a goofy math course and the idea has waxed and waned in popularity over the years, it's a viable way to plan meals—*big* meals.

I love those magazine stories extolling the virtues of Volumetrics by showing two photos side by side. In one picture, there's a dense little cube of fudge surrounded by vast expanses of empty dinner plate. The fudge is delicious, but in one or two bites you've consumed enough calories to feed the population of Botswana, and you've still got most of the dinner hour ahead.

For the same number of calories you can have the heap o' stuff that's on the second plate in the second picture—egg-white vegetable omelet, slabs of whole-wheat toast sparkling with butter-substitute spray, mounds of fruit and vegetables, baked apples with cinnamon, bowls of steaming soup. You'll be eating what's on that plate till next Tuesday, but the fudge sinker is long gone, a distant burp.

With Volumetrics, you plump up your portions with high-volume, low-density foods, the kind that naturally contain a lot of water and fiber (soups, vegetables, beans) that make them bulky without adding much fat. The presence of fat *always* means caloric density, because fat has more than twice the number of calories per gram (9) than either protein or carbs (they both have 4).

It's not a bad way to learn how to put meals together. Pasta with marinara sauce and grilled chicken can be "diluted" with vegetables. Come to think of it, nearly any dish can be improved with fruits or vegetables.

Add mandarin orange slices to salad. It's like meal extender but without breadcrumbs.

I'm never going to calculate every stalk of celery or shovelful of roughage I ingest. I don't want to be that precise or tally figures on spreadsheets every day. My general aim is to get the most satisfaction on the fewest calories and to feel like I've had a *meal*. You can find tips on how to do that—add volume to your meals without adding fat—on the Mayo Clinic website (www.mayoclinic.com). One suggestion is to begin lunch or dinner with broth-based vegetable soup; by virtue of the time it takes to eat it (especially if it's really hot) and the volume inherent in any soup, you're less hungry for the rest of the meal.

Even when an eating plan is sound, try not to get hooked on it to the exclusion of all the other good-sense advice out there. You should get information the way you get nutrients—by grazing widely.

Case in point: The Glycemic Index is worthwhile information in small doses (especially for diabetics, the only ones who really care that much about blood sugar). But there are people who build a shrine to the Glycemic Index, and while genuflecting there they miss the bigger picture. It's true that some foods raise (and then drop) your blood-sugar level more dramatically than others, but just because ice cream is low on the G.I. doesn't mean it's healthier than carrots, which are way up there. A baked potato, as nutritionally perfect a food as you'll find, practically has a red warning slash through it on the Index.

If it seems that there are hundreds of ways to lose weight, and that 99 percent of those ways are gimmicky, it's because there's mad money to be made in the weight-loss industry. How else to account for the popular diet book *Eat Right 4 Your Type* and its numerous offspring, which advise that you eat specific foods depending on your blood type?

Dieters *love* gimmicks. They're driven to them because gimmicks are zingy and capture the imagination. Fads fill a need even when what they're pitching isn't necessarily healthy. If a particular diet or nutritional philosophy grabs you, then—and I say this guardedly—even a crackpot diet might be worth it as long as it helps get you started.

But there are not really hundreds of ways to lose weight. Reliable studies prove that most diets eventually lead to low-fat, limited-calorie plans masked as something else. Even the low-carb eaters tire of their hunks of meat and gradually move toward taking in fewer calories.

It cannot be said enough: You can lose weight initially on *any* diet, no matter how off-the-wall it is. The key is whether you can go on to make the transition to sensible eating, which *always* requires a reduction of fat and calories (or an enormous increase in energy output) no matter how you spin it.

If you're determined to try a commercial diet, then you've *really* got to eat right for your type. And what type might that be? If you're a perfectionist who likes to make lists, there's Weight Watchers, where keeping track of points can give you the rush you normally get from filing documents in triplicate.

If you have the ability to hyperfocus on one massive project at a time yet can't seem to match your socks, the imposed structure of a diet might be just the tonic. Many of them—like The Zone and Jenny Craig—offer prepackaged meals that relieve you of the burden of making dining decisions. (But remember, it's expensive, and you can't use that crutch forever.)

If you want to lose weight but you're not ready to give up certain things, you could go on Atkins (but not if you have a heart condition or high cholesterol), where you get the semblance of being at an all-you-can-eat buffet.

If you lack focus and you're social, join a meeting-based plan, like TOPS (Taking Off Pounds Sensibly), Weight Watchers, or Overeaters Anonymous. If you lack focus and you'd rather bleed from the eyes than mingle with strangers, do an online program where you can learn at your leisure at 3 A.M. in total seclusion.

My cousin Anne, a religious Christian—long story—followed a faith-based diet where I presume Jesus was counting the calories on her behalf. It didn't work for long, but then Jesus probably has better things to do.

As a rule, no one stays on any one plan forever, not even when it carries a divine stamp of approval. Commercial plans are designed to appeal to the broadest segment of society, and as you know from hotel bathrobes and hospital gowns, one size never fits all—or "most," as they coyly phrase it these days. It's no wonder these diets have recidivism rates estimated at north of 95 percent.

It almost doesn't matter which method you choose—even the Phases of the Moon diet might have something for you—as long as you end up eating the way you're going to eat for the rest of your life. You've reached your goal not when the scale hits the sweet spot but when you embrace the behaviors it will take to keep it there.

And what are those behaviors? You won't find them listed in the books with the groovy titles. More people will buy *Eat Your Way to Thinness with Pork Rinds!* than a sensible, dusty tome like *Watching Paint Dry: Lose Weight the Slow, Boring Way!*

Integral to my weight loss was how long it took—two and a half years to lose 75 pounds. I actually began to recoil when people advised me to step up the pace. I *wanted* my body to adjust gradually. I wanted my head to adjust at the same rate. Every time I'd lost weight in the past, the minute I received unwelcome sexual advances I'd rush home to eat. I suppose the two-letter word *no* would have been more effective, but for a host of reasons as tangled as the ones that made me sneak candy as a child, the word *no* was not in my vocabulary. Instead, I was stuck on Plan A: *Get fat and you won't have to deal with saying no.*

Slow weight loss—you've heard of it. But you don't believe it. Or maybe you think you—*and only you*—can get around it somehow. I have a friend whose husband mainlines coffee; he grudgingly admits that coffee contains caffeine and that caffeine has been proven to increase agitation. But—he insists anxiously, hands vibrating—he *alone* is immune to the effects of caffeine. It doesn't interfere with his sleep—this said at 3:30 A.M. when he was up and puttering around. No, his cellular makeup is biologically different from that of all other humans.

Slow weight loss is for others, not for me . . . so says the pre-contemplative, vestigial reptilian brain located in your spinal cord.

It has somehow seeped into the public consciousness that a person can lose 10 pounds a week. Every week. I'm here to tell you: It won't happen— unless you're planning to check yourself into a WWII concentration camp. Running a marathon, which is 26.2 miles, eats up approximately all the calories in . . . *one pound of fat.* You'd have to run a marathon every day *and* cut calories to lose 10 pounds a week. (Yes, your metabolism would increase, but not to warp speed.) Even though Helene reported back from her first marathon that there was a Ghirardelli chocolate station about a mile from the finish line, which makes me contemplate a career in long-distance running after all, if you wind up eating more just because you're burning more, then you'll have an even *harder* time losing unrealistic numbers of pounds per week.

The calories in/calories out equation is true in the abstract, although there are other factors, such as how efficiently your body burns fuel. The bottom line is that people are generally not active enough to burn 10 pounds, or an extra 35,000 calories, a week. Starving yourself won't do it, because once the body senses starvation, the whoop-whoop alarm goes off and your metabolism goes on its own little hunger strike, conserving energy to make it as tough to lose weight as it is to pass a Fifth Avenue co-op board. With your metabolism on slowdown, the minute you start eating normally again your body lovingly protects its new store of fat, clutching it like Scarlett O'Hara caressed her turnip—*"As God is my witness, I'll never go hungry again!"*

The shred of truth that makes people think this kind of dramatic weight loss is possible is that during the first week of any diet the numbers are impressive. Never mind that it's mostly water, not fat. If you ate salted popcorn last night and got on the scale this morning, you know what I mean; your weight can fluctuate 5 to 7 pounds from day to day just from how much water you retain. Losing water weight is meaningless in terms of weight loss except for the undeniable psychological boost.

Quick weight loss is neither feasible nor desirable. Study after study confirms that slow weight loss is more likely to last. Chuck all the nonsense the advertisers feed you and the false promise of the new diet your best friend swears by. Instead, learn to be thrilled with the considerable accomplishment of losing one to three pounds a week.

Or less.

A reader wrote in to complain that I wasn't "serious" about weight loss because I was losing so slowly. One of my editors buttonholed me to complain, "Enough with that one-pound-a-week bullshit. That's a joke."

But it's no joke. Unable to sift fact from fiction, so many people assume that the jury's still out on how to lose weight. But the jury weighed in decades ago and hasn't changed the verdict: Successful weight loss depends on eating a variety of foods in moderate portions, with an emphasis on low-fat and whole-grain, adding fitness, and losing weight slowly while making behavioral adjustments.

There's wiggle room, tricks that make incremental differences, such as foods that metabolize faster, fine-tuning meals according to nutritional density (as in Volumetrics) or the proportion of nutrients they provide ("food combining"), and theories on how best to strengthen muscle, which burns more calories even at rest and takes up less space in the body (that's why you can appear thinner without necessarily losing weight).

They've recently nailed down scientifically what everyone's been saying all along, that breakfast is the most important meal of the day. (Most of the thirty or so people who faint each month on the New York City subway system are weight-conscious young women who skipped breakfast, according to the Transit Authority.)

Research yields new information every day on appetite hormones and how fat and diet intersect. But health professionals haven't changed their tune about the *basics* of weight loss, no matter how many fad diets have come and gone, no matter how many carbs have been sent to the gulag. Just because the average consumer is confused by information overload doesn't mean there's doubt among people who study the subject and aren't trying to sell special government-suppressed vitamins on the side:

- Eat healthfully and plan meals ahead.
- Control portions.
- Move vigorously.
- Change your lifestyle in ways you can sustain.
- Set realistic goals ("I want to be Kate Moss without the coke habit" is not a realistic goal).
- Put some education under your belt instead of crème brûlée.
- Stay mindful.

It's not always simple to put all this together. Neither is it confusing. Although there are healthful properties in red wine and dark chocolate, no one at the Mayo Clinic is recommending the Merlot Diet or that candy bars replace an apple a day. As they proclaim at the University of Wisconsin Eating Disorders Clinic, "Live a reasonably healthy lifestyle, and accept the body that results."

If all those professionals seem to know the key to lasting weight loss, how come you haven't been taught the secret handshake?

The information is out there, not hidden, not government-suppressed. Here's some one-stop shopping: the National Weight Control Registry that began in 1997 with 784 participants. To enroll in the NWCR, subjects had to have lost at least 30 pounds and kept it off for a year. It didn't mat-

⭐ The Stylist: Dorian May

I never thought I'd see the day when I'd march into Bloomingdale's and say, "No thanks, I don't need help. My stylist will be joining me shortly."

New York magazine named Dorian May the best personal shopper of 2004. But that's nothing compared to a recommendation from Amanda the Exercise Nazi. When I needed several perfect outfits in a hurry for a photo shoot for the front cover of this book, Amanda sternly told me this could *only* be accomplished in the company of Dorian. Now that I've worked with her, I see why. This Paris-trained stylist "preshopped," then helped me choose seven sexy, lovely outfits so the photographer would have lots of options.

"Are you okay?" she asked when she noticed me turning ashen in the dressing room. It wasn't because I didn't like the clothing, or even the price tags. After more than a dozen years of trying to hide my body under dark colors and baggy clothes, it was a thrilling yet frightening thing to allow myself the possibility of a stylish, colorful, form-fitting wardrobe. It took some getting used to.

The world of clothing had changed since the last time I wore a size 12. I felt like Dorothy after the tornado, stepping across the threshold into a wonderland of color. Dorian guided me through gowns, wrap dresses, and halter tops; among sequins, sparkle, and asymmetrical hemlines; and past wedge heels, patent leather, and leopard print. I practically needed my asthma inhaler in order to cope.

Is it too chichi to have your own stylist, even for just that once? Not if it teaches you to stop buying basic black in voluminous sizes and thinking of your body as something to cover instead of enhance.

ter how they lost the weight, just that it be a substantial amount that didn't come back to them like spit in the wind.

In fact, this particular group had lost and kept off an average of 66 pounds apiece.

The authors of that first Registry research paper, published in the *American Journal of Clinical Nutrition*, looked at what these people had in common. How did they do it? What was the hallmark of their success?

They found that no matter how long the subjects had been fat or how many diets they had tried, "nearly every participant used diet and exercise to initially lose weight, and nearly every subject is currently using diet and exercise to maintain his/her weight." No big surprise so far, except that 42 percent said that maintenance was *easier* than expected.

In follow-ups and as more people joined the Registry (you can too, if you qualify), researchers isolated what set the success stories apart from the heavy hordes who tried and failed. What makes some people so special?

- They eat breakfast. Independent research points to breakfast eaters consuming fewer calories later in the day than they would have if they hadn't been fortified by a bowl of cornflakes. A seemingly conflicting report had it that breakfast eaters consume *more* calories, yet are less likely to be overweight. In any case, everyone agrees that a healthy breakfast is a good thing. Calorie bargaining ("I'll skip breakfast and eat more later") doesn't work.

  The NWCR research also found that breakfast eaters have more energy and burn more calories during the morning.
- They try again. It took an average of seven attempts before they got it right, meaning that every failure brought them closer to success.
- Tortoise beats hare. Those who eventually gained a few pounds back were likelier to have lost weight too quickly at first, or to have had more problems with portion control.

- They keep their eyes on the prize. Regainers got sloppy and let their gym memberships lapse.
- Calories count; low-fat rules. No matter how they lost their initial weight—half on their own, the other half through regimented programs—"maintenance of weight loss is associated with continued consumption of a healthy low-energy, low-fat diet." All roads lead to portion control and reducing fat intake.
- The longer you do it, the easier it gets. This is *really* good news—"risk of relapse seems to decrease over time." Success breeds success, and no, you won't have to obsess and count calories every second of every day into your dotage.
- They changed their eating *and* their physical activity. Not just one or the other.
- They love it. They all learned to love exercise, low-fat eating, and the feeling of power that weight maintenance confers. Note that they didn't necessarily start out that way. They didn't say, Hey, I want to get up before dawn and jog on a lonely highway! But they couldn't help it—healthy living is wildly infectious; you can come down with a case of it for life.
- They didn't play fast and loose with the rules. I know people who are "good" all week and allow themselves to go hog-wild on the weekend. But the research found that those who were consistent with what they ate "were 1.5 times more likely to maintain their weight within 5 pounds over the subsequent year than participants who dieted more strictly on weekdays."

What does the NWCR tell us? It's all good. It's easy to grasp. The people who screwed up were the ones who didn't trust the basics, who got fancy or lost focus.

Another giant ongoing study bears out the NWCR findings and adds a few of its own. The Nurses' Health Study, begun at Harvard Medical School in 1979 (with another phase added in 1989), started out with 122,000 nurses who were interrogated regularly over the years about their diet and health. This was more than a "How're ya doing" kind of questionnaire; the nurses submitted 68,000 sets of toenail clippings, don't ask me why.

Although it was originally designed to look at the long-term consequences of taking oral contraceptives, the Nurses' Health Study amassed a wealth of information on weight loss.

You know how they always say married men are healthier than bachelors? Good for them. But a 2005 paper found that divorced women had lower body mass indexes than married or remarried ones. They were more physically active, too; a 1994 paper showed that "higher levels of activity were associated with better cognitive performance." Ladies in lousy marriages, call your lawyers.

The study also concluded over the years that being fat "predicted a higher risk of death regardless of the level of physical activity" and that yo-yo dieting meant "greater weight gain, less physical activity, and a higher prevalence of binge eating."

So there you have it. Trustworthy information isn't always the warmest and fuzziest. That's why the most popular diet books, wanting only to assuage the reader, tend to be of dubious nutritional merit—from today's *Eat Right 4 Your Type* all the way back in history to *No More Alibis*, which was No. 1 on the *New York Times* best-seller list of 1934.

The author of *No More Alibis* was billed as Sylvia of Hollywood, aka Madame Sylvia, a beauty columnist for *Photoplay* magazine. She was considered an expert in her day simply because so many women read her, a tautology that still exists: If a diet book is a best-seller, it must be right. Right?

No matter that Madame was horribly misguided on just about everything she advised. For better posture, have a friend slap you hard on your back to remind you to stand up straighter. The leg exercises (there are pictures!) are actually for the abs. The abs exercises are for the birds.

The caption for Figure 11 advises, "Use your hands to squeeze off fat on the calves." That's from a section on spot reducing, which we now know is impossible (although you can firm up the underlying area by building muscle).

The stretches Madame extols would probably slip you a disk. And she admonishes, "Don't swim if you are fat, it will only develop you more." She also claims you can get rid of a double chin by slathering cold cream in upward strokes.

It's quaint and funny. But have things really changed? I've gotten countless e-mails assuring me you can "lose weight while you sleep!"

I must admit that Sylvia of Hollywood had one sensible bit of advice: "Get up and dance about the room, sway and swing to the music of a snappy fox trot!"

Living healthfully is a technique, not a torture. That's what the *real* experts say.

FOOD

check my calendar often to see what my work schedule is like the next day, the next week, the next month. I can't just get out of bed any old time, stretch lazily, scratch my butt, and then find that I was supposed to be at the new Adam Sandler movie half an hour ago.

Yet that's how most of us handle food—haphazardly. Meals are an afterthought. Or no thought at all. Just when your hunger is reaching epic proportions and the growling in your stomach is frightening the neighbors, you realize you have no idea what's for dinner. Is there even any food in the house? You could make a nice healthy vegetarian Boca burger with a salad, but you don't have any Boca burgers, you don't have any salad.

How about an EggBeaters omelet? No eggs, no beaters.

There's canned soup, but you can't wait the full two minutes for the microwave to stop churning; you're too hungry by now.

Wait, you have dinner fixings on hand after all—a menu for takeout pizza, a telephone, and a finger for dialing!

⭐ Think Different

Chef Terry sez: Nothing to eat in the house? Take a closer look. Hmmm, frozen chicken, old cans of soup . . . Try thawing the chicken, cutting into chunks, then browning and tossing into the soup. Simmer until the soup's reduced by half. Ladle over brown rice.

What's this, an old box of cornflakes? Crunch it up, season it, press seasoned fish fillets into it, lay fillets on lightly greased sheetpan, add some liquid like lemon and wine, bake about 8 minutes at 350.

Not everything labeled "burger" has to be served on a bun. Take salmon burgers: Fry 'em up, julienne the patties, add to penne pasta tossed with canned diced tomatoes. Add canned peas and a bit of parmesan.

If a can of asparagus is not so old it needs to be buried, resurrect it by draining and rinsing the contents, then purée it in a food processor with garlic, tarragon, salt, pepper, and a pinch of cayenne pepper. Heat as a sauce to use over fish or chicken.

Healthy eating requires forethought, especially if it's a foreign concept to you. You don't have to preplan meals down to how many pinches of oregano in the pasta sauce, and you don't have to lose sleep over Wheat Chex versus Rice Chex. But you should have a general idea of how your next few days are shaping up: How many nights you're eating home, what groceries you need, which freezer-burn mystery packages need defrosting, and an approximate date for when the leftover milk will congeal into a foul pudding.

Does it make sense to pack lunches this week? If so, is there a pita pocket in the house, perhaps under the sofa cushions? Should you whip up a batch of chicken salad with dried cranberries and apples (watch the mayo) on Sunday so you'll have some Tuesday? Should you freeze half a pot of chili or vegetable soup in small portions for emergencies?

What about desserts? When 10 P.M. rolls around, you'd better have something small and sweet on hand or there'll be trouble. There's nothing more depressing than driving to the 24-hour supermarket in bathrobe and curlers, waving an ax: *Outta my way, I need a sugar fix!*

Chef Terry's Guide to a Comfortable Kitchen

DISCARD dull knives, rusty peelers, ugly mugs you wouldn't be caught dead drinking from, and all food whose expiration dates passed with the last gold rush.

KEEP only what you need—and that's less than you think. A kitchen can function with just four knives and four small implements. The knives: 8-inch chef's knife, paring knife, thin boning knife, slicing knife. The implements: peeler, sharpening steel, strainer, box grater (which can shred, slice, and grate). Knives go in one drawer (or in a countertop wood block), small tools in another.

SPEND on good pots and pans. For pots, you need a 4-quart, an 8-quart, and a 12-quart. For pans, you need a 7-inch, a 10-inch, and a 14-inch, each with a lid. They should all be heavy and lined with copper, clad in stainless. Get the expensive stuff; it lasts a lifetime.

You need one more pan for stews and braised foods called a sauteuse—usually 12 to 14 inches in diameter, double-handled, about 3 inches deep, with a lid. To store, I slide the lid over the handle of the appropriate pot or pan, then hang the pair together from a hook.

I was never comfortable in the kitchen. Mom didn't like anyone in there when she was preparing dinner. She was relatively new to kitchens herself and therefore nervous if anyone watched her, a casualty of her own mother's restrictions on company in the kitchen. Mom was sent out to work full-time when she was sixteen, and she handed over her paycheck (except for cigarette money) to her parents; no time for learning to cook. Forget the terrors of young brides on their wedding nights and imagine instead the kitchen virgin who suddenly has to cook for husband and, eventually, children. My father came from a family of food lovers and food pushers, so the pressure was on. Mom was expected to cater to my dad (the baby of eight) and pick up where Grandma Annie had left off.

The first time Mom tried to make hamburger, she didn't know about defrosting. She hacked at the giant frozen brick with an icepick, then clattered it into a frying pan and inadvertently discovered "black and blue," where meat is crisp on the outside, raw inside. There was a long learning curve, during which she didn't welcome us kids underfoot.

Diane and I were largely left to our own devices for breakfast. We even packed our lunches; I remember making my bologna sandwiches when I was six because Mom worked days and Dad worked nights.

Our breakfasts devolved from sugary cereals (Cocoa Puffs, Lucky Charms) to cake eaten off a paper towel and soda straight from the can. Dinner remained a family affair, but anxiety was the chief condiment; Diane's chair was nearest the kitchen and she'd rise with her fork like a vampire to swoop down on the choicest pork chop before anyone else could get to it, adding to my sense of food deprivation (*The best piece is gone!*). Mom liked to watch the six o'clock news while we ate in silence. I was sometimes sent to my room without dinner for giggling.

Breakfast was more exciting than dinner anyway. Who needs a nasty ol' pork chop when you can have Entenmann's cake left over from dessert the night before? With no one to say no, we'd carve ourselves ever bigger slabs of it: yellow sheet cake with gooey chocolate frosting, crumb cake with granular sugared outcroppings, and the treat of treats, "blackout layer cake," its layers conjoined with pudding-like frosting, jet-black and sensuous. There was a cookie crumble on top like a dusting for forensic fingerprints.

So I never learned to cook. I made a few unspeakable attempts in my first apartment, an Upper West Side brownstone studio with a roach problem. I learned to eat out a lot.

Every now and then I'd get a homey urge to fill the kitchen with lovely aromas. There was that muffin-baking kick when one day, reason unknown, it occurred to me, Wow, how about if I were the kind of person who baked muffins? I immediately bought a how-to book, filled my shopping cart with every ingredient for the muffins on display in the book's glossy pages, and proceeded to make batches and batches. The most labor-intensive were the apple-cinnamon, the most pleasing the chocolate cream cheese.

This was back when I didn't have a weight problem, although it was an indicator of one in the making.

I couldn't eat *all* of them, of course, even though they were mini-muffins. So I packaged them individually in aluminum foil and crammed them into the freezer like the Tribbles on *Star Trek*. For a week or two a defrosted, reheated muffin was a treat, even though, unlabeled, I was as likely to get a cranberry as the highly valued chocolate cheesecake. Then, like Tulipmania in 1630s Netherlands, when tulips were in such demand they became more expensive than houses and the bubble finally burst, I got sick of all the muffins and they became worthless iceballs interlocked tightly in the freezer like soundproofing.

The muffins lay there for months, perhaps years. They thought they'd discovered Ötzi, the mummified Iceman, in my freezer, but it was only a blueberry muffin. Each time I went for ice cubes, a few dense muffin balls would thud to the linoleum floor.

I still have the mini-muffin pans, though I never used them again. They join the ranks of specialty equipment I've amassed over the years for hobbies that burst out of nowhere and soon receded—all the gear you'd need for horseback riding, for example. The day I bought those tight riding pants with the leather reinforced crotch I knew I was in trouble, because usually a large outlay of cash toward equipment is the day I lose interest in the activity. (Actually, I didn't lose interest in horses; it was just too expensive. My last riding instructor said I had "a good seat," and I'll always treasure that, whatever it means.) Overspending and overeating are linked, coming from the same places of emotional need.

I still think from time to time, Wouldn't it be lovely if I were the kind of person who baked muffins *and* rode horses?

But I digress. To lose weight, you have to cook for yourself. There's no way around it. Restaurants undermine you with hidden oil, butter, salt. Did you ever wonder why takeout Chinese food stays so hot even though when *you* steam vegetables they cool off immediately? Because the restaurant adds *hot oil* before the container leaves the premises. Ever wonder why those mashed potatoes are so creamy and delicious at the corner bistro? Because they're *drowned in butter and cream!*

Homegrown Condiments

Chef Terry sez: I'm getting away from store-bought condiments, which are heavy on oil, salt, and preservatives. Instead of brand-name pasta sauces, I use cans of diced tomatoes mixed with fresh herbs and a tablespoon of olive oil. Instead of store-bought salad dressing, I fill a bottle with quality olive oil and balsamic vinegar, plus Dijon mustard and herbs . . . and shake. That becomes my base dressing, to which I can add ginger powder and a bit of teriyaki sauce—even some tomato juice for "tomato vinaigrette."

When I was between apartments, I stayed with my friends Terry and Diane. Terry, you will recall, is a chef. The first time he cooked for me, he piled our plates so high I couldn't see either my of hosts across the table. Terry was just doing what chefs do.

"Uh, Terry, these portions are a little large," I ventured, not wanting to bite the hand that overfeeds me.

"Really?" he said, looking as blank as my cat Buzz after he's peed in the cactus plant. *Really? Did I do something wrong?*

The next time Terry plated my food, the mound was slightly lower; I could just make out the chandelier over the rice pilaf.

I was spending too much money and too many calories at restaurants and from takeout food. So I took a series of cooking classes at a school for chefs across the street.

I loved it. Watch me mince garlic!

In the first series of lessons, a remedial course for people who get panic attacks if they're in a kitchen for any reason other than to locate the pile of takeout menus, I learned to make frittatas. I made almost as many frittatas as I had mini-muffins during Tulip-muffin-mania. I'll never make a frittata again—the thought makes me nauseous—but I turned out some damn fine specimens in my frittata prime. (The key is to dot the top with goat cheese right before finishing it under the broiler.)

Flush with frittata success, I moved on to bananas flambée. Soon I was teaching Amanda's children, Charlie and Evan, how to tilt a ladle of rum over an open fire, catch a flame on its fumes, and pour the dancing blue blaze over a concoction of butter, cream, and brown sugar. Oh, and bananas. I just know that Amanda was delighted to see her children playing with fire at the stove; how quickly they grow up!

I graduated to a series of French cooking lessons where pretty much all you learn is how to make cognac-cream sauce from pan drippings. The teacher was brutal; I've never seen someone so angry as when she witnessed a student putting a "savory" next to a "sweet" on a plate. But every week she was back with an all-new lesson plan: "Today, class, we'll be making cognac-cream sauce. Next week, something new: cream with co-gnac sauce. And butter."

I eventually took a spa-cuisine class. But when you're first learning to plan meals, keep it simple. Know your ingredients. You can't go wrong with oatmeal for breakfast, it's made of . . . oatmeal. You can see what's in a salad topped with grilled chicken. Once you start getting fancy, you lose track of just what and how much went into that dish. Turkey breast on whole wheat is simple. Chicken potpie is not: What's in the glop? What's under that crust? Why are you eating puff-pastry crust anyway?

Roger Ebert's Perfect Rice-Cooker Oatmeal

Roger has a weird fascination with rice cookers. For all I know he makes pot roast in them. He lost a lot of weight by walking with a pedometer and starting each day with his own rice-cooker oatmeal:

Begin with good pure oatmeal, no preservatives or flavors or sweet-eners. Plain Quaker Oats are fine, or get organic. Add 2.5 cups water per cup of oatmeal. Chop and add fruits of choice: Apple, pear, banana, berries, raisins, prunes, kiwi, whatever pleases you. Optional: One table-spoon ground flaxseed. Must be ground freshly (grinder, or mortar and pestle) or it will pass through undigested. Optional: Cinnamon (good with apples or pears).

Combine ingredients in rice cooker. Turn on. The rice cooker does the rest.

You don't want to court boredom, but if you need the comfort and structure of a small, revolving menu of favorites, shake it up just enough to keep the old favorites interesting. If omelets meet your seal of approval, play around with what you put in them—different vegetables or herbs, for example.

You might think the solution is to hock everything and hire a personal chef. *Wrong.* You've got to learn to feed yourself, not only to save money and evaluate what you're eating, but for the sense of mastery and self-nurture. Prepared meals and takeout are temporary, stopgap solutions.

⭐ Chef Terry's Food Facelift

Familiar foods can get a facelift without expensive plastic surgery:

Cucumbers: Peel, split, and seed them, then cut on an angle to get away from the tired old cuke-circles look.

Leafy greens: Julienne them so they mix better when tossed with cut vegetables.

Carrots: Rough-cut those sticks at different angles to break up the monotony of a single shape.

Cheese: It's a bit whimsical, but you can use a star-shaped cookie cutter when adding cheese to a salad.

I'm not Oprah Winfrey. I can't afford a full-time chef. But as the Incredible Shrinking Critic, I was able to command a meeting with Donna Mintz, a vivacious chef and former fashion designer who goes into people's kitchens, cooks up a batch of healthful, balanced meals for the week, and packages and labels them with simple instructions for getting them to table.

I found Chef Donna at her website, www.basilandbarbells.com. I cleverly timed our meeting for when I felt I was slipping off the rails.

Chef Donna unreasonably refused to hand over her database of 1,000 healthy recipes even though I flashed my press pass at her like an arresting officer, but she agreed to share these tips:

- Figure out meals the week ahead and shop over the weekend.
- On Sunday, prepare side dishes and marinades for the protein, package them in portions, and store them in the refrigerator (for no more than four days) or freezer.
- Wrap the protein tightly and store. Cook it on the day you eat it, reheating sides and sauces. Dinner in 20 minutes!
- When packaging food, use the smallest possible container. The less air, the better.
- Thaw frozen food overnight in the refrigerator.
- Eating doesn't have to be repetitive or uninteresting; change it up.
- Use only the freshest ingredients.
- Stick to low-fat cooking techniques: sauté, roast, grill, or steam. Use nonstick cookware and as little oil as possible. One millisecond spritz of cooking oil is all you need.

I put Chef Donna's advice to work when my mother was in too much pain from arthritis to cook for herself. I'd fix Mom a week's worth of meals, all packaged in portions and ready to freeze. It gave me an opportunity to experiment in the kitchen, and I'd siphon off half of what I cooked for myself.

Preparing and apportioning meals in advance made a huge difference. My eating habits stopped their temporary free fall and *my mother gave me a compliment*—several, in fact. The vegetables in balsamic reduction were a particular favorite.

It was cheaper to eat this way, too. Overspending is cousin to overeating, so if you rein in one, it's likely you'll rein in both. The trick, as always, is follow-through. I couldn't very well chain Chef Donna to the radiator and make her call out recipes whenever I needed inspiration. Fortunately, there's Google, a tool that has many uses aside from getting aerial photographs of celebrity homes. If you Google "low-fat chicken recipe" you get 3,400,000 results; that should tide you over for a couple of dinners.

Brite Bar's John Libonati

I was heartsick when my neighbors John Libonati and Chris Schutte moved away. John's a chef, now owner of Brite Bar in Manhattan, who used to hand me special hors d'oeuvres and drinks over our adjoining patio fence. The new neighbors don't hand me *anything* over the fence. Bastards.

Before moving away, John shared some of his cooking tips for cutting fat and adding flavor:

"I'm all about substitution, an easy way to kick up flavor. Substitute low-sodium chicken stock for water, or add fresh herbs to foods being blanched, poached, or boiled. When making rice, I use half water and half low-sodium chicken stock; you don't have to add butter or anything else. Works great with brown rice, too.

"I was about to make a cassoulet, but Chris freaked out over all the duck and duck fat in the recipe. So I substituted olive oil for the duck fat and used chicken stock when cooking the raw beans.

"Don't throw out those squeeze bottles of Dijon mustard or low-fat mayo. Add chopped fresh herbs, plain yogurt, and a dash of balsamic vinegar with a bit of olive oil and shake. You now have a low-cal salad dressing (plus you recycled without even trying!). These are also great for taking on picnics or to the beach, and the dressings are great over raw veggies.

"For cocktails I dilute flavored vodkas with soda water. If they seem bland, ask the bartender for a lime or orange slice. When ordering a mojito, ask the bartender to skip the sugar. Also look for Bacardi's half-the-carbs rum. Don't be afraid to bring your own low-cal cranberry juice to a holiday party."

Out of curiosity, I Googled a few simple dishes to see if there'd been any improvements on them since last I boiled water for pasta. This is how I learned that soft-boiling an egg was an art (let it warm to room temperature first to avoid cracking) and that the answer to that conundrum about whether to pour cold water over cooked pasta to remove the starch or not to pour is—*not* to pour. It makes it harder for the sauce to stick.

You can lose weight whether your eggs crack or your pasta is runny. But cultivating the habit of trawling for recipes, nutritional information, and kitchen hints helps keep you focused on the goal of nurturing yourself. Many's the time I've stared at my groaning pantry—jars of capers, sacks of pine nuts, eight-packs of crushed tomatoes—thinking, Gee, there's nothing to eat here. Now what I do is Google "low-fat recipes capers." (Only 115,000 results this time; ah, here's a Turkey Stew from the Dominican Republic!)

Googling whatever's in your pantry for recipe ideas is one way to get past that "there's nothing to eat" feeling.

When I stayed with Diane and Terry, I saw how Terry invents meals on the spot. He stands in front of the open refrigerator, gazing, gazing. Like Thumper, he taps one foot rapidly, unconsciously, while he calculates his options. At his restaurant where he works, he has to plan methodically, but at home he grabs food off shelves like a mad scientist and combines them in creative ways, crumbling Boca burgers into the pasta for a low-fat Bolognese effect, adding herbs to grated parmesan cheese.

If that's too casual, you can begin by deciding on a main dish, then build side dishes around it.

But don't go crazy. I remember dining at a typical steakhouse in Austin where the portion of meat was the size of a small child. Alongside it, like a Stonehenge slab that had keeled over, was the biggest, longest, heaviest baked potato I've ever seen. Both meat and potato drooped wearily over each end of the long plate, artifacts from the radioactive wake of the

Nevada Test Range. If you looked closely, you'd find a tiny sprig of parsley nestled between them; the salad, I presume.

Needless to say, that's *too* much protein, *too* much starch, and not enough vegetable. Yes, a potato is technically a vegetable, but along with corn and peas it's so starchy it passes for bread.

★ Threesomes

Chef Terry sez: To make a meal as appealing as possible, the finished plate should have a trio of complementary colors, like the pale neutral of fish with red sauce and a green vegetable. The same concept applies to a trio of contrasting tastes—Asian cooking often juggles sweet, bitter, and salty. Another prossibility is a trio of textures, such as pasta (soft) with sugar-snap peas (crunchy) and diced salmon burger (chewy).

To get an idea of what a healthy dinner looks like, check out the visual on the website for the American Institute for Cancer Research (www.aicr.org) under their "New American Plate." Less than a third of the plate is devoted to animal protein (although it won't kill you to eat vegetarian on occasion), while most of the plate goes to vegetables, whole grains, beans, and fruit. Personally, I'd give grains slightly less than a third of the dish, and keep fruit separate as a planned daytime snack or a dessert atop a scoop of sorbet. (Pomegranate on sorbet is ambrosia.)

Dinner doesn't have to be exotic. A small grilled steak or spice-rubbed piece of salmon is fine.

The spa-cuisine class taught us how to make fish in parchment paper. When you wrap the fish (loosely) in the paper, topped with vegetables and a bit of white wine, the warm air from baking makes the paper puff up like a balloon. Inside, the fish steams. The dish is healthy, fun, and impressive for guests, as if you've wrapped them a little present.

But I'm not trudging back from late-night screenings only to julienne carrots and crimp parchment edges. Movie critics, believe it or not, do *not* get free popcorn, a popular misconception. In fact, the projectionists who run the critics' screening rooms don't allow us to bring in *coffee*; they peer at us through their peepholes and storm in if someone rattles a Ricola. When I get back from a hard day at the mines without sustenance, I'm ravenous. The only recipe I want to see is "Cut slit in plastic overwrap, place in microwave."

★ Building Blocks for Quick Meals

Chef Terry sez: My cooking is based on a series of building blocks. For what I like to call the "Costco Kitchen," I need only four items for the main-dish building block: A lean red meat, a fish, a poultry, and a pasta. Each item will later be prepared two or three different ways, giving me a dozen different meals from one shopping trip.

Also when shopping, I buy things with a long shelf life for stocking the kitchen. I get chicken or turkey sausages packed in Cryovac, as well as frozen Boca burgers (they're vegetarian) and salmon burgers. I get canned goods like green beans and chickpeas for adding to dishes and salads. I pick up interesting spice mixes and seasonings to rub on meat and fish— although I also make my own Chef's Superspice with salt, pepper, garlic powder, onion powder, cumin, and a pinch of cayenne and paprika.

When you get home from shopping, immediately apportion the main items before opening the refrigerator. I divide the chicken into two bowls. One gets a sprinkling of Superspice, then stored individually or two pieces at a time in freezer Ziplocs (push out the air from the top as you roll them up). The other soaks in a marinade of teriyaki, ginger, and lime juice. I julienne a few extra breasts to use another time as a quickie stir-fry or to sauté and add to pasta.

Salmon freezes well. A few portions, 4 or 5 ounces apiece, get a dry-rub mix of Superspice and dried dill. Other portions get a marinade of my basic salad dressing, to which I'll add ginger powder.

The trick is to spend the time up front preparing food for fridge and freezer so that no time at all is needed when you have to get dinner on the table. I have it down to thaw, then broil, bake, or sauté. It's a no-brainer.

Example: Thaw fish, throw in pan, add can of diced tomatoes and juice of one lemon plus some dry-herb mix, heat till it simmers, and finish under broiler for 3 to 4 minutes to brown lightly. Serve with vegetables and brown rice.

On these occasions, Lean Cuisine and Amy's frozen burritos are perfect. And I'm in love with my George Foreman grill. The little "cookbook" that came with it is a riot—every recipe is a variation on: *Marinate the meat. Put it on the grill. Serve and enjoy!* You want a steak? *Marinate, grill, enjoy!* You want fish? *Marinate, grill, voilà!* There's nothing you can't marinate and grill on that thing—meat, vegetables, pineapple slices. *Bon appétit!*

★

All the meal planning in the world won't help you lose weight unless you factor in reasonable portion sizes.

Like the old joke—Of course I can give up smoking, I gave it up twice this morning!—I lost weight on Weight Watchers several times. (And gained it back.) But it wasn't all for nothing, because their "points" system—the bane of many a dieter—gave me an early solid idea of portion control. Without understanding servings and portions, you're sunk. A serving of rice or pasta is half a cup, which is what fits into an ice-cream scoop. Pathetic, I know.

WW is constantly retooling the points system to make it easier and less "points"-like. But it's still a handy bit of knowledge, a shorthand alternative to adding up every single calorie in the day. The goal is to learn to eyeball servings and portions effortlessly—and yes, there's a difference between "serving" and "portion." A serving is a basic unit of a food, as in, "eat 3 to 5 servings of vegetables a day." A serving size of a vegetable is generally half a cup. If you have 2 cups of vegetables on your plate, then you have one *portion* made of 4 servings; a portion is what you actually put on your plate, and it's a quantity that usually bears no resemblance to serving sizes.

In any case, don't make the mistake of calling a wheel of brie a "serving" when that is a "portion." Also, a doorstop.

What works better for me is the cheat sheet you can download and fit in your wallet from the National Institutes of Health (they suggest you laminate it, a precursor to bowing to it), where servings are described in terms of everyday objects. There is the old familiar deck of cards (or the size of your palm), which is approximately three ounces of meat or chicken. A music CD is a pancake—not a pancake I've ever seen, admittedly, more like the *idea* of a pancake. But technically a serving size of pancake all the same.

Ping-Pong ball: two tablespoons of peanut butter. Checkbook: fish (you get five to six ounces of fish per day if you choose that as your protein, versus three to four ounces of chicken or steak). Bar of soap: cornbread.

Is there someone who sits in a dark room thinking these things up? A hockey puck equals one of those small Lender's bagels. A 9-volt battery is your cheese quotient. The NIH describes a serving of fruit, ice cream, rice, or pasta in terms of half a baseball. Serving sizes must have been invented by men, hence the sports analogies. A hockey puck means nothing to me and I'm not bringing one in my handbag should I ever get a table at Lutèce. But I get the drift: A serving of bread is the size of a cassette tape, not the loaf of challah it takes two waiters to hoist on their shoulders.

Portions have ballooned in the last twenty years. The National Heart, Lung, and Blood Institute has a "portion distortion" slide show with side-by-side pictures of what we ate then and what we eat now—like the simple, no-frills cheeseburger that was 333 calories in the olden days and 590 calories today. You'd have to lift weights for an hour and a half to make up for the difference in calories between those two burgers. A typical plate of spaghetti has more than doubled in the same time, from 500 calories to 1025.

If you're looking to avoid housework, taxes, or just about anything else, nothing beats calculating your daily caloric intake using the various charting tools you can find online. It'll take all day! You won't even have *time* to eat!

No one was more surprised than I was to find that the government offers a really useful website for that purpose, www.mypyramidtracker. gov. It's laborious, but after you enter your daily food intake and physical activity, it generates wonderfully detailed charts about exactly what you're doing with and to your body—how much selenium you took in, for example, in case you were wondering. If you get a frowny face next to your abysmal attempt to meet the fruit requirement, a pop-up instructional tells you what you're doing wrong and how to fix it. (Hint: *Eat more fruit*.)

It's an excellent educational and motivational tool. But the real lure is that it creates the kind of busywork that dieters crave as they monitor their progress.

The site has its peculiarities. The fitness tracker, which wants you to account for all 24 hours of your day, has no entry for writing a movie review, but there are entries for "orange grove worker" and "steel mill: removing slag," and one category that integrates "forklift operator" with "yoga instruction." Not since Jennifer Beals in *Flashdance*—welder by day, exotic dancer by night—has there been such an intriguing job combo. Under "home activities," the limited choices include "butchering animals" and "cooking Indian bread on an outside stove"; I'm happy to try just as soon as I remove some slag and get my degree in forklift/yoga.

Calories aren't the whole equation. Nor are percentages. If you're getting only 25 percent of your calories from fat, that's wonderful, but not if you're meeting that percentage by upping the overall intake, as per the SnackWells Syndrome. Yes, olive oil, nuts, chocolate, and wine have healthful properties, but two tablespoons of oil are 240 calories, and when they say "eat nuts" they mean five ounces per *week*, not per TV program.

Often you're damned by your own quest to "eat healthy," because foods are so cleverly marketed. The FDA should demand asterisks on every health claim so the fine print can read "Mr. Health's Tar for the Veins snack packs aren't really healthy, and Mr. Health's name is actually Fred." You can't blame corporations for wanting to maximize profits. But you have to keep sight of your obligations as a consumer to read nutritional labels, choose carefully, and take your sweets with a grain of salt, or you'll be adding useless calories to your day.

Take Jamba Juice, a new chain that's colonizing the nation the way Starbucks once did. I see them everywhere now selling fresh-squeezed juice drinks, some with added ingredients like yogurt or sorbet. We all know that fruit is healthful and most people never get enough of it, so if you have a fresh-squeezed fruit drink it's better than no fruit at all. But juice drinks are deceptively caloric, especially if you're gulping it to quench your thirst. At least Jamba Juice has actual fruit in their drinks, as opposed to supermarket products that are nothing more than sugar-water, a waste of calories when you could have bitten into a nice, juicy, fibrous orange.

Just as at Starbucks, you have to order carefully at Jamba Juice. A Starbucks Frappuccino is a *milkshake*, and before Starbucks came along you probably never considered having a milkshake before noon. Some of Jamba Juice's "smoothies" are likewise milkshakes, even if they contain vitamins.

The Jamba PowerBoost—which their website hails as "all about SU-PER nutrition!"—has 570 calories of super nutrition in the largest size. The "100% pure orange juice" in it is the "health" come-on, but the ingredients also include "jamba sorbet," which sounds to me suspiciously like dessert.

The "blended" drinks are somewhat lower in calories, but an Açaí Eye-Opener, despite being "infused with guarana, soymilk, strawberries, and bananas," plus a hit of caffeine for starting the day, is 430 calories in the "Power" size of 24 ounces. (The "Original" size has 350 calories, still a lot of calories for a glass of juice.) The Power-sized Sunrise Strawberry is 540 calories, thanks to soymilk, nonfat plain yogurt, frozen strawberries, and frozen bananas. You get the picture.

A famous *New York* magazine cover story once exposed breakfast muffins as being loaded with calories. Just because it's "lowfat" (or marketed as breakfast food) doesn't mean it's not a 650-calorie bomb. "Lowfat" foods usually supplement the taste with extra sugar. Conversely, "low-carb" foods supplement with fat. The claims on the packaging purposely don't tell the whole story.

Don't be dejected. Being a food cop can be exciting, like finding a quarter in a pay phone. Or finding a pay phone. Many food chains post their nutritive stats *somewhere*, even if it's on a website you have to click through creatively to get anywhere. I enjoy ferreting out the information and turning the act of being a responsible consumer into a treasure hunt.

If you're whining that someone should just tell you what to eat, then you're going to have a difficult time in life, and not just in losing weight. My sister and I grew up with the nagging feeling that we had no idea how to take care of ourselves. We were right. So now we're learning. You can't be a baby bird forever, screaming in the nest with your beak open for predigested worms to be spat down your gullet.

To eat healthfully you need to know what you're eating, and for that you need to look at food objectively. Run it through a mental checklist:

Just because a bran muffin has bran, is it "healthy"? How many servings are in it? What's the story with the add-ons, like Cinnabon's cream-cheese frosting? Am I eating this because I believe it's good for me when maybe it's not? Is it the only food option I have at this moment? Will I feel better or worse after eating it? How will it help me achieve my long-term goals? Does Cinnabon offer extra cream-cheese frosting on the side? (Yes, it does. But Devin Alexander offers an amazing recipe in *Fast Food Fix* for shaving 371 calories off a homemade Cinnabon.)

Yes, portion size is a runaway train in America. Food here is cheap and abundant, government subsidies have made corn syrup and its variants the main ingredient in our diet, and ad campaigns underscore our national obsession with getting our money's worth (*Now, with more! Extra! Biggie size!*).

Fast-food franchises continue to seek to top one another, even while giving lip service to "health" by offering salads (which are sometimes higher in fat and calories than burgers), and even though McDonald's nervously withdrew its "supersize" menu right before the debut of the documentary *Super Size Me,* in which filmmaker Morgan Spurlock ate nothing but McD's for a month and got so fat and sluggish his doctor begged him to stop killing himself.

Spurlock got the idea after a particularly big meal. "I was sitting on my mother's couch in West Virginia, all Thanksgiving'ed out, the Al Bundy hand-in-my-shorts thing, tryptophan in my veins," he told me after his film debuted at the Sundance Film Festival. "I was watching TV and they had on those girls who were suing McDonald's for making them fat. Where do you draw the line between personal and corporate responsibility? McDonald's says this food is healthy and nutritious. Well, if it's *that* good for me, I should be able to eat it for breakfast, lunch, and dinner."

On Day Two of his eating plan Spurlock upchucked his Happy Meal from the car window. And as the weeks ticked by he became fat, depressed, and a lousy lay.

But he persevered, newly addicted to salt and fat, traveling our great nation in search of regional differences. "Oh my gosh, the McDonald's Texas Homestyle Burger, it was great! They also have a McRib in certain places, a monstrous concoction, basically a ground-up pork sandwich pressed into the shape of ribs. The barbecue sauce makes it bearable."

His girlfriend, a vegan chef, was repulsed.

After thirty days, Spurlock's cholesterol was "off the charts." His blood pressure was "awful." "I was depressed, exhausted, and my doctor said my liver was basically like pâté. My sexual energy was kaput. I could have slept 15, 16 hours a day. Garbage in, garbage out."

There's one thing fast-food joints could do to improve, says Spurlock: "Make a veggie burger that doesn't taste like ass."

Spurlock, whose film was nominated for an Oscar, may have single-handedly halted the "supersize" juggernaut. But the term was already in our vocabulary and in our blood, like the manifest-destiny doctrine of the settlers who kept heading west for more and more land. There was no such thing as too much land. Now there's no such thing as too much chopped meat. How else to explain Hardee's Monster Thickburger at 1410 calories and 107 grams of fat? It's an assemblage of two $\frac{1}{3}$-pound slabs of beef, four strips of bacon, three slices of American cheese, and an untold amount of mayo, on a buttered toasted bun. It's 600 calories more than a Whopper with Cheese, more than twice the calories of two Big Macs.

All for less than six bucks.

Jay Leno joked that it comes in a cardboard box shaped like a coffin. The Center for Science in the Public Interest called it "food porn." The Hardee's ad campaign: "If you want more meat than this, you'll have to buy a hunting license and a rifle."

The food critic of the *Chicago Tribune* called it "unfortunately delicious."

When I was in junior high, I discovered that I could stretch my weekly lunch money if I ate two Scooter Pies and a Coke instead of buying the school lunch, which was no garden of healthy eating itself. The money I saved went to a worthy cause: ice skating. I learned that Scooter Pies and soda made a perfectly acceptable bargain lunch.

We live in a fat culture. Food is everywhere, larded with fat and salt, always within nostril range, offering financial incentive, with hundreds of variations on burgers and shakes and creamy coffee drinks and snacks.

Renée Zellweger was paid $3.5 million over her salary to put on a few pounds; that buys a lot of Monster Thickburgers.

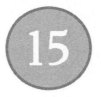

EXERCISE

There's a rock two-thirds of the way down the slope of a particular run at Deer Valley Ski Resort in Utah. Every time I took that run I had to take off my skis, unbuckle my boots, and sit on that cold, sharp rock for 20 minutes because my feet would ache so badly I couldn't continue. The base lodge was within sight; even the poorest skier could make it there in three minutes. Not me. Never me.

One time after sitting on that rock I hailed a snowmobile ski patrol as if it were a taxi. "Are you hurt?" asked the driver skeptically. He was accustomed to broken bones and arms hanging from their sockets, not some fat chick who can't face the final few yards en route to an après-ski hot chocolate.

"I'm *exhausted*," I said as if I'd just dug myself out of an avalanche after three days gone missing.

Even the thought of Deer Valley's famous turkey chili couldn't get me

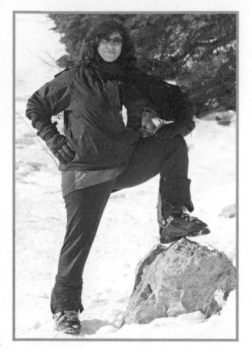

The Rock at Deer Valley. *(Photo by Steve Wilson, courtesy New York* Daily News*)*

down the mountain without a pit stop at my rock. I didn't have the excuse of bad rental equipment, because my boots had been custom molded to my feet and secured by red buckle extenders—blazing red so that everyone on the slopes could share in the knowledge that my feet were too fat to buckle into ski boots the normal way.

I had no illusions of becoming a great skier. Good would do. Even fair was fine. But these modest goals were a long way off, since I seemed to suffer from a rare ankle ailment from which there was no respite except a rock on a hill.

The ankle ailment magically cleared up the minute I lost weight. When I returned to the same slope 50 pounds lighter and with months of squats and lunges on my side, my rock—quite literally my touchstone—was just another unremarkable piece of landscape as I whooshed by. Three minutes to turkey chili!

In a surprise move, I took up skiing relatively late in life as part of my postcancer splurge on lessons of all sorts. There were kayak lessons and horseback riding lessons. I finally learned to drive. And there was skiing. I must like the turkey chili at Deer Valley a lot, because skiing requires all the things fat people hate—extreme temperature, lugging and schlepping, wearing form-fitting clothes.

You need a month with a personal trainer just to carry the equipment. Renting skis is much like a visit to the DMV, involving standing on line

⭐ Readers: The Hiker

Jim Feher walked off 70 pounds by hiking near his home in Dingmans Ferry, Pennsylvania. His motivation? Being measured for a tux for his brother's wedding. "After years of accusing my wife of shrinking my clothes in the dryer, the truth was finally revealed," he says. "Hiking is an awesome way to get in shape and lose weight and inches. When I hike I can eat four meals a day and snack and still keep the weight off."

and shuffling from station to station where small, seemingly insignificant tasks are accomplished. There's one station just for judging what pole length you need. A cute ski stud who couldn't be more disgusted with his job holds several samples near your armpits; he eyes you, then the poles, then you again, and shakes his head sadly. They'll let *anyone* ski these days, he seems to be saying.

But there's a wonderful shopping opportunity in the world of ski gear. If specialty catalogues are anything to go by, you need twelve layers of clothing of different weights and fabrics and wickibility. You need a jacket with hundreds of zippered pockets, so that if you ever *did* need your asthma inhaler while aloft on a chairlift, you'd be dead before you found which compartment you'd stuffed it in.

You don't just need gloves and socks—you need liners for them and liners for the liners and warmers for inside the innermost liner. There are clever hooks on the jacket from which to hang necessary items. Your ski pass, of course, which the chairlift attendant inspects with suspicion as if you might be smuggling contraband. Also, dozens of indispensable items that need hanging from those hooks, like ChapStick, goggles, antiglare lens wipes, locker key. The cherry that tops it all off is a knit hat from which flow mock Rastafarian braids for that special fat-white-chick-reggae look.

⭐ Readers: The Jumper

"I decided to lose at least 60 pounds and so far have lost 10 with eating right and exercising. I really want to recommend a great exercise—my son begged me to do it—and that is jumping on a rebounder! [A portable trampoline.] On it you can walk, jog, do jumping jacks, jump rope, all to your favorite music."—F.H., VIRGINIA

Putting on ski boots is impossible, buckling them exhausting, walking in them unthinkable. No matter how many layers you wear, you'll freeze, except when you're in a sunny spot sweltering. This is not a sport that attracts fat people, especially when you factor in that there are no cute ski outfits in their size. The most effort they'll agree to make is to draw their own hot chocolate from the spigot.

It's not laziness, although I know it looks that way. Fat bodies are designed to conserve energy, protect the precious store of fat. When I was fat I rarely felt like jumping up and doing a jig, yet once I lost weight and went to the gym I began to relish—yes!—running up the stairs. It's still me, the same person, neither better nor worse. There's hardly an exercise (aside from carb loading) that will get a fat person off the couch voluntarily—which is why when you take up exercise, it's got to be something you absolutely *love*. Or at least something you remember loving at some point. That's one of the keys to a fitness program: Go for something you loved as a kid.

I love skiing because I love snow and just want to be near it. I love horseback riding because of that old "Black Stallion" fixation that figured so prominently in my childhood diaries.

I always loved riding a bicycle. When I got my first two-wheeler, "Blue Lightning," I had a dream that it was a horse and that I rode it in the playground to the astonishment of the second grade. In my twenties, I

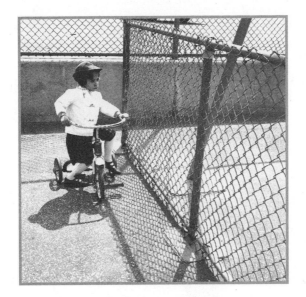

My first horse . . . er, tricycle.
(Photo by Sam Bernard)

lived steps from Central Park, where I'd bike a few laps almost every day. When I moved to a neighborhood without any greenery, the bike simply took up precious real estate in my apartment until Jon and Helene moved in down the hall. Helene has a picture of herself from when she had an astonishing six-pack, and now she's on a ruthless quest to regain that impressive musculature by any means necessary. She bought a kiddie carrier for her bike, plopped Nick in it, and roped me into riding with them up and down the newly revamped West Side bike path bordering the Hudson River. It's a beautiful run, but narrow, so that much of the ride is spent screaming at pedestrians who don't realize the path belongs to those of us on mighty two-wheeled steeds.

The first time I went riding with Helene and her toddler, she was so excited for the company that she pointed out the sights along the way—families fishing or picnicking by the water's edge, an ugly Trump high-

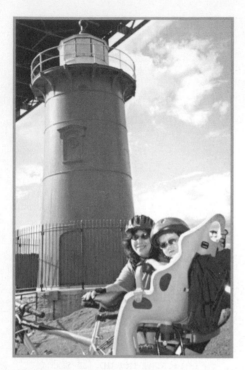

Me and Nick at the Little Red Lighthouse.
(Photo by Helene Rutledge)

rise on its way to blocking everyone's view. I followed Helene's pointing finger and ran my bike into a curb; I squeezed the brakes on both handlebars in a reflex gesture and went ass over teakettle. It's not fun being the fat person on the ground. I was so stunned by this sudden turn of events that I hyperventilated, felt sick, and had to sit on a park bench with my head between my knees while Helene flagged down passing cyclists in an attempt to score me a sip of water.

My body's reaction to the fall said it all: I wasn't fit. I couldn't hide it. A fat person astride a bike has some credibility, but the same fat person unable to cope with a simple fall and too shaky to continue is fooling no one.

This bike incident took place before I lost weight. Even after, cycling didn't always go smoothly. Another time on the West Side path Helene and I tied up our horses at a railing near the Boat Basin and I lost my famously Balanchine balance—my foot was caught in the saddle—toppling not only *my* bike but also the entire railing with all the other bikes chained to it. Nick was still sitting in his kiddie caboose and over he went.

I'm not fit. I'm clumsy. I'm a menace to public property. And now I'm a child abuser.

Nick was fine. I plucked him from the hedge he'd fallen into. His baby helmet had slipped over his eyes, but he was leaning placidly into the

★ Readers: The Walker

"I decided it was time to take control, and so far, I've lost 27.5 pounds. I do not have a personal trainer. I walk on my treadmill—which I know is boring, but it works for me." —T.C.

prickly hedge, probably assuming this was all just part of the magical world of adult activity.

Eventually Helene (and Nick) and I would do 10-mile bike trips up the path to the Little Red Lighthouse under the George Washington Bridge, a landmark made famous by a children's book. Getting there was a great feeling of accomplishment, despite that scene from *In the Cut* where a maniac slashes Meg Ryan in the lighthouse and she has to walk miles back down the bike path, all bloody, not a single car picking her up. (If she'd had gigantic breasts, *someone* would have taken her, blood and all.)

When I was fat, I wouldn't "exercise," yet I was happy to go biking. If only we could call exercise something less terrifying and prescriptive. Perhaps we could call it "transcendence," as in "I think I'll put in a sweaty hour of transcendence this morning, honey, it's so uplifting!"

Fat people don't want to move because their bodies don't want them to. There's also the embarrassment factor: who wants to be the only one whose clothes fit poorly, who huffs and puffs, who falls off the bike and gasps like a landed fish? To forestall such iniquity, fat people resort to a range of excuses that usually includes *I don't like exercise.*

But there's no one who exercises regularly who doesn't love it. Their bodies crave it like a drug. "I'm like a bag of jingle bells!" JoAnne fretted one day when it was raining and she couldn't work off stress by running across the Brooklyn Bridge with her husband.

⭐ Phil Campbell

According to Phil Campbell, author of *Ready, Set, GO! Synergy Fitness,* the "Holiday Seven"—those seven pounds people purportedly gain during the holidays—is a misnomer. "Most people gain less than one pound during the six-week period between Thanksgiving and New Year's Day," says Campbell.

But fat people typically gain five pounds. Campbell blames Metabolic Syndrome X (ooh . . . so *Blade Runner!*) It's a cluster of symptoms involving the body's insulin resistance, and it usually coincides with extra abdominal fat, higher cholesterol, and weight gain. The afflicted don't process food adequately, which makes it easier for them to gain weight.

The cure for Metabolic Syndrome X is, unsurprisingly, exercise and eating a balanced diet.

The drug analogy isn't far off the mark. Exercise floods you with endorphins, the substance you get from chocolate—which explains why chocolate is to Valentine's Day what gold, frankincense, and myrrh were to the Christ child. The stereotype of lonely ladies eating bonbons in bed, there's something to it.

Technically, endorphins are polypeptides that bond to neuroreceptors in the brain to protect you from pain. They're responsible for "runner's high," that jolt of euphoria that'll knock your athletic socks off if only you can stick out your aerobic routine for 15 or 20 minutes. When I'm cranky, I like to tell myself (sometimes, admittedly, with no discernible effect): *You're only 15 minutes away from bliss.*

The endorphin rush is free. It's legal! And it's almost better than sex—the "almost" because sex *also* releases endorphins.

There's more to it, of course. Among other things, exercise:

- Is the number one predictor of success in long-term weight management.
- Builds muscle, which keeps burning extra calories even while you sleep. (Is that what they mean when they advertise you can lose weight while you sleep?) The engine burns hotter for about 45 minutes after stoking it with a heart-pumping workout.
- Restores all that calorie-burning muscle you otherwise gradually lose as you age.
- Keeps you strong, supple, and happy.
- Makes your clothes fit better.
- Deflects the progression of osteoporosis by keeping bones strong.
- Staves off a variety of illness and disease and helps you recover from them faster even if you do get sick.
- Sends oxygen to the brain.
- Helps you lose weight and feel proud of your body.
- Opens up new spending opportunities at specialty sports stores.
- Wards off dementia, according to the latest research. (If you're having trouble remembering this one, then you aren't exercising enough.)
- Makes it legitimate—cute, even—to wear sweatsuits.

These are just some of the widely known benefits of exercise. There's no downside once you get over the hump of getting off your ass.

Physical fitness comes in three flavors: stretching, weight-bearing activities, and aerobic exercise. Doing something is always better than doing nothing, but the goal is to have all three of these flavors in your daily diet.

Easier said than done; I hate stretching. It's probably because I was never very limber—another genetic predisposition. When the class instructor tells us to sit with legs spread and reach forward to stretch the back and the hamstrings, I use peripheral vision to check out everyone

⭐ Fidgeting

People who fidget expend an extra 350 calories a day and tend to be thin, according to the *New York Times.* That can account for losing 40 pounds in a year. Are certain people genetically inclined to fidget? If so, does fat interfere with their urge to fidget, or are nonfidgeters prone to fat because they're naturally more sedentary?

else—they're gracefully touching their foreheads to the high-gloss gym floor. Can you say *murderous rage?*

Stretching feels good if someone else is stretching you, which doesn't happen often enough in life as far as I'm concerned. If someone else wants to bend me and twist me, fine. It's when I have to do it myself that I sulk; I find it mostly tedious. That's why I was so happy to hear about an ongoing controversy in the field of stretching: some exercise physiologists say it's useless, if not downright harmful. Fred Hahn, author of *The Slow Burn Fitness Revolution,* argues that flexibility is a function of genetics and muscle strength, not endless, painful attempts to force the body to go Gumby. There's research in the field to support this (as well as research showing that eating protein is better protection than stretching for reducing postworkout soreness). Hahn says that the reason you can reach farther at the end of a series of stretches is that the pain of the stretches cranks up the endorphin machine, sending out a natural opiate like a lullaby. The endorphins mask pain, and absent the warning signs of pain you can push your body beyond where it really wants to go.

Hahn uses as an object lesson the common case of aging ballerinas who overstretched so much during their dancing days that their shoulders and knees pop out of joint at will, ligaments dangling like a marionette's strings.

But there's stretching and there's stretching. If you have problem areas, you should stretch them. It took a long time for me to realize that the point of touching your toes isn't actually touching your toes or trying to get your wrist or your elbow down there without bending the knees. The point is to stretch the lower back. Stretching teaches you about your body and keeps you limber; if you rarely move your arm, you're liable to get the aptly named "frozen shoulder."

Here's what most professionals agree on when it comes to stretching: If it hurts, you're overdoing it. Don't stretch a "cold" muscle (get the blood circulating first). Learn to differentiate between "real" pain (a sprain) and "exercise" pain (the buildup of lactic acid, which gives you an almost pleasurable muscle ache); the difference is clear once you've experienced the lactic-acid scenario a few times and begin welcoming it like an old friend.

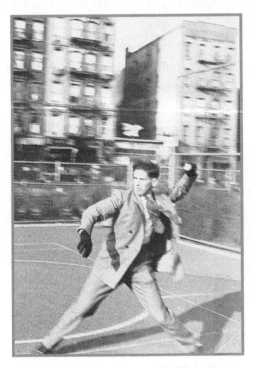

The second type of physical fitness involves weight-bearing exercise. A muscle gets bigger and stronger only when it's worked so hard it suffers microscopic tears (as cruel as that sounds). The body takes some time to lick its wounds and make repairs—which is why you shouldn't work out the same muscles two days in a row—and pretty soon you're Jack LaLanne, pulling tugboats in the water by a strap between your teeth!

Are there still women out there who think that lifting weights will turn them into steroid freaks at

Daddy playing handball on the Lower East Side. He loved displays of strength and agility.

Muscle Beach? Personally, I'd *love* it if I could make a bulging muscle pop from beneath smooth, streamlined arms, like Nessie rising to the surface for a rare photo op. But it's not going to happen. Because of men's innate body composition and various hormonal influences, there's no way women can compete (without drugs) in the bulging-biceps arena. You can pump iron till your arms rip off and leave bloody stumps, as in that *SNL* skit about Eastern European power lifters, and you *still* won't have what they have. (Was Freud wrong? Was it not the penis women were after, but a set of trapezius muscles that would make our necks look like souvenirs from the redwood forest?)

It's too bad some women still fear weight-bearing exercise, because women in particular need it to forestall the effects of age and menopause, which rob us of estrogen and calcium, leading to weight gain, increased risk of hip fractures, and the overall specter of osteoporosis. Even if you didn't drink a lot of milk when your bones were growing, it's not too late to strengthen the muscles, and there are so many ways to do it.

You can use free weights, weight stacks, or stretchy bands in Day-Glo colors. You can do it with ordinary household furniture or by holding a jar of olives in each hand. There are ultraslow, nonsweaty workouts (Fred Hahn's Manhattan studio teaches the "slow burn" method), and there's nonstop circuit training that mixes in cardio with the weights. Body-sculpt classes at gyms are just as effective as having a personal trainer. You can use fancy equipment or no equipment. If you're extremely heavy, merely walking can be considered a weight-bearing exercise.

The one thing to watch for is proper form. Without it, you can hurt your back, strain your neck, or miss getting any benefit from the exercise whatsoever. Walk around any health club and you'll see people arching their backs when they shouldn't, hunching their shoulders to help a nearby muscle that's struggling, lift themselves into a sit-up through momentum instead of contracting the abs, or using weights that are so light the muscle isn't challenged.

⭐ Readers: The Boxer

"I lost the most weight when I had a trainer at Gleason's Gym in Brooklyn. I did three rounds in the ring with a cop once. My trainer was from St. Thomas, and when he screamed at me, 'Use your job! Your *job!*' I yelled back, 'I'm a *writer!*' Finally, I realized, halfway through the second round, that he meant I should use my 'jab,' not my 'job.' After that, my boxing improved."
—JEREMY KAREKEN, NEW YORK

The third area of physical fitness is aerobics, or cardio. Anything that gets your heart rate up and that you can theoretically sustain for hours fits the bill: jogging, biking, swimming, running to steal someone else's cab. It doesn't matter what you do as long as you pump oxygen through your system, but not to the point where you can't hold a conversation. You might think the goal of doing aerobics for an hour a day is preposterous, but start with 10 minutes, three times a week and see what comes of it.

Of the three flavors of fitness, aerobics is best at burning calories, and they burn most efficiently when you're *not* at top speed. That's why, once again, brisk walking (where you're slightly out of breath) is to exercise what the baked potato is to food—simple, balanced, perfect.

I was fortunate enough to sample some expensive fitness programs and equipment while researching my column. But fancy is as fancy does. I was offered a free trial membership at the Sports Club/LA, a fitness emporium described by *New York* magazine as "the purest expression of gymness ever built." It was *such* a pure expression of gymness—a temple for the truly rich and thin—that I went only once. There's such a thing as too much gymness.

You don't need to spend a dime to get in shape. There's nothing you can do at a luxury gym that you can't do at home. You can get a full toning workout from feather-light, ultrapackable stretchy bands. They're also helpful for stretching. A small set of handheld weights and a mat and chair are all the tools you need at home; even just the mat and chair will do. A jump rope for aerobics, how much can that set you back? The key to exercise is making it interesting and fun, not spending on fancy gear. You can spring for a ThighMaster or you can lie on your side on a mat and do leg lifts; a tight budget isn't a valid excuse for skipping exercise.

The biggest rationale for not exercising is that you have "no time," which really means "no time for *that,* but plenty of time for other stuff." Do you mean to say you don't have 15 minutes in your entire day that you can spend bopping around your living room to music?

The second-biggest rationale is that you don't have the energy. Not surprising, since energy begets energy. That's not some Far East philosophy, and it's simple to test: Rev up for a few minutes, get breathless, and see how great it feels. If you can commit to starting out with 10 minutes a day for exercise—*10 minutes!*—then at the end of that 10 minutes you probably won't mind adding an extra 5. And so on, as you build up stamina.

★ Energy Bars

"Energy bars"—candy bars in disguise, but with less taste—get their attractive-sounding name from what the Center for Science in the Public Interest calls a "labeling loophole." Strictly (and legally) speaking, all it means is "calorie bar."

There's a story my family likes to tell about me, probably not as a compliment, about the time I decided one scorching August day to learn to jump rope. I went out to the shadeless concrete playground (no Evian bottles back then) and practiced with a chartreuse plastic jump rope with yellow handles, jumping jumping jumping in the hot sun. For hours. Until I got it right.

Mania? I call it passion. My goal wasn't just to learn how to jump rope but to jump it faster and better than anyone else in second grade. I got so fast the jump rope became a faint chartreuse blur, a protective iridescent bubble around me. Did you know you can shave seconds off your time by not really *jumping*, but merely lifting your feet a fraction off the pavement?

Today, decades later, I occasionally have some of that can-do spirit of childhood. But I sure as hell don't have the stamina. I took a pop health quiz in the September 2004 issue of *Prevention* that promised to rate how much "boundless energy" I have— mentally, physically, emotionally. I didn't have any, at least

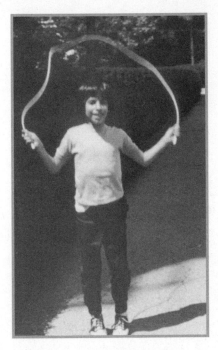

The chartreuse plastic jump rope.
(Photo by Sam Bernard)

none you could point to as "boundless." The last time I had energy like that was when my grandmother was yelling at me across the playground, *"Don't run!"*

When I was fat, my top walking speed was three miles per hour, which felt like the fastest a human body could possibly move. After about six months doing the treadmill a couple of times a week, there came a day when I unconsciously broke into a sustained run—well, a slow jog— even though I hadn't expected ever to run again in my life.

It felt like I was racing across the sky.

16

BEHAVIOR

During a stopover on a Caribbean cruise, Marie led me on a jaunty walking tour of Old San Juan. I usually have trouble keeping up with her because of her preternaturally long legs—I refer to her apartment as the Land of the Giants because she and her husband keep the snack foods on shelves I can't reach—but this time it wasn't her stride that was at fault. I could barely go a few yards without having to sit on the curb, because for months, my left heel had been growing gradually more sensitive to the slightest pressure.

"You're walking like an old lady!" snapped Marie.

Old lady? Hadn't she seen the pictures of me running the L'eggs Mini-Marathon? The minute we got back to New York, I marched—okay, I hobbled—to the podiatrist. It would be six months before I could get out of sneakers.

"Does my weight have something to do with this?" I asked the podiatrist.

She peered over her glasses. "It surely doesn't help." She did a mathematical computation in her head to determine that every step I took added something like a billion pounds of pressure per square inch on my heel. Walking when you're fat is like pounding your feet with a mallet.

How do you get the horses back once they've left the barn? With plantar fasciitis, there's no one method guaranteed to work, but there are several options: Physical therapy with electrodes, as if my foot were starring in *Manolo Blahnik's Frankenstein*. Stretches. Custom orthotics that squeaked, announcing my decrepitude with every step.

Last stop: Cortisone shots— which, the podiatrist assured me briskly, are *extremely painful*.

Running a Corporate Challenge race in Central Park.

None of these options made the slightest difference on their own, so I tried them all. The podiatrist, that vixen, was right—the shots were painful! But she told me something that stuck: To get to the tipping point, sometimes you have to try everything at once.

So it is with losing weight. When you're twenty, you can *think* about weight loss and it'll happen. As you age and you have more weight to lose, and your body is reluctant to give it up (*Mine!*), you need to unleash a strategy of shock-and-awe—hit it with everything you've got. That's

243

every technique and trick you ever learned about managing food, maximizing metabolism, getting help, staying focused, and fine-tuning where possible.

★ Readers: The Strategist

"After many years of struggling with controlling my weight, these are some of the practical things I've learned: You have to move and you have to sweat. Choosing what I eat is the determining factor in how I make the exercise work for me. Substitution is one of the basics; you can give up ice cream for soy yogurt and candy for fruit, keeping in mind it *does* get easier as you go. Grazing is another way of eating, with the rule of thumb that you don't eat more than what will fit into your two cupped hands in a three-hour period." —G.E.

You need to do all of it, whatever it takes, in some combination and to the highest degree possible, building up to it gradually until you reach the tipping point. Cutting calories is a start, but it's not enough.

When you combine several techniques like this, it's hard to stay focused after the initial flush of success. Just as you need physical fitness, you need *behavioral fitness* to keep yourself on track. Here's a sampling of some behavioral techniques you'll need:

Goals

Make them specific, not "I want to lose weight." Don't peg your goals to other people's perceptions or make them semantically slippery. Goals need to be succinct and measurable, spanning various aspects of weight loss, including exercise and behavior: I will walk for half an hour, five times a week. I want to see my blood-sugar numbers fall below the prediabetic zone. I will eat before I go shopping, so I'm more likely to stick to my grocery list.

In the case of my reader Irwin, he wanted to live to see his grandchildren.

Goals can be phrased negatively ("I don't want to go up another size") or positively ("I want to run a marathon"), and you need a range of them to suit fluctuations in your needs and mood.

My goals included: I don't want to wear clothes that hide my body. I want to tuck a shirt in. I don't want to be the fattest person in gym class. I want to be able to do twenty push-ups, and not the girlie "modified" kind, either. I don't want to be out of breath when I run to make the light. I want to fit within the molded contours of bus seats so that the seat next to me doesn't remain suspiciously empty during rush hour. I want to feel good after eating a meal.

I don't want a recurrence of breast cancer.

My most cherished goal, the one that was most honest and resonant for me: *I want my body back*. I didn't fantasize that I'd be seventeen again. There are scars. I've aged. I accept that nothing will be precisely as it was. There probably won't be many offers of free pizza for life.

Still, I wanted the return of my body, the one I recognized as mine, the one I was proud of, the one that felt sexy. The body I jumped rope in and rode bicycles with as if they were horses. I danced in that body, *lived* in it, and dammit, I wanted it back!

My other goals were reasonable and true, but the goal that really gets you going isn't always the one that sounds noble or that meets other people's expectations. "I care about my health" is a lovely sentiment, but if your true motivation is to make people at your high-school reunion jealous, well, you're not the only vain, superficial person on the planet. Go for it.

These goals by and large aren't numbers. True, I was inspired by the idea of losing 100 pounds. People reacted with alarm, thinking I couldn't possibly have that much weight to lose. But I always knew that in the end I'd accept a healthy weight, one where I felt at home. *Thin* to many people means "boyish," and I haven't looked boyish since I wore braces. I've come to see *thin* as stringy, ropy, haggard. Not a look I crave.

Making goals out of clothing sizes is deceptive, because sizing has become as elastic as the waistband on my Fat Pants. Marilyn Monroe, symbol of sex appeal and vulnerability, famously wore a size 14—the same size that today we'd probably call a 10. Sizing has changed over the years, first as a way to flatter the wealthy into thinking they could fit into couture dresses that were retooled for them off the runways. But why should only the rich be cosseted by the clothing industry? All women's sizes have morphed over the years to soothe our fragile egos. After I dropped down to 170 pounds, I fit into a few size 12s, depending on designer and cut, but size 12 is what I remember wearing in my early thirties, when I weighed 135. Seems like 8 is the new 12.

Clothing size, though highly motivating to many, doesn't tell the whole story. A fit person can slide a smaller size over her tight muscles than a person of the same weight who isn't fit. Aiming for a particular size isn't specific enough for the many goals you want to set (and for which you want to reward yourself when you achieve them). Here are a few more goals I set myself one New Year's Eve:

I will put my fork down between bites. I tend to clutch my fork throughout the meal like Charlton Heston at an NRA rally with a rifle at the ready; "from my cold, dead hands!"

I will write fitness appointments on my calendar. That makes it official. When you say, "Hey, let's you and me hit the gym this week," it's like saying, "Let's do lunch!" You don't mean it. You can wiggle out of it. On my calendar program I have "Gym w/Diane" as a recurring weekday event at 7 A.M. Even when I don't make it, I still have to stare at those words on the computer screen; I can't very well claim it slipped my mind.

I will re-up my subscriptions to nutrition and fitness newsletters. They're fun to read and keep me focused on health. They always throw in a tidbit I didn't know, like which tantric position burns more calories.

I will try to do "the plank" for 60 seconds. Contrary to popular belief, I do have abdominal muscles—you just can't see them. A six-pack appears only after you've lost enough body fat to make them pop. I have abs, yet I can't seem to master that exercise where you hold yourself up on your arms and your toes, back straight, in the push-up position. After 30 seconds I retreat into the "child's pose" of yoga, where you look like you're bowing obsequiously to royalty.

I hate the plank, but I aspire to 60 seconds of it anyway.

I will make my closet look like Amanda's. My size-zero friend Amanda the Exercise Nazi keeps her wardrobe pared down to essentials plus some high-quality items for special occasions. In the past I never knew what size I'd be from one full moon to the next, so I amassed tons of clothing toward which I felt indifferent. The closet was packed and depressing, prelude to a panic attack. In Amanda's closet there's *space* between the hangers.

I will snack between meals. Nothing kills resolve like heading into the home stretch for dinner with a raging appetite nipping at your heels. Whatever good eating I've done all day doesn't count if I blow my resolve on one meal where I overestimate my nutritional needs (*"I could eat a horse!"*). A small healthy snack between meals is prophylactic medicine.

I will clean off my desk. Just kidding.

Reminders

Prevention magazine suggests putting a mirror on your refrigerator—not to scare you but as a reminder that you are what you eat. A snapshot of you will do, or a healthy-foods shopping list.

What *not* to have on your refrigerator: The magnet for Domino's Pizza delivery.

I'm not the sort of person who looks in the mirror and recites a daily affirmation: "Who loves ya, baby?" I'd rather drink hot coffee from my cupped hands than from a mug that says "Today is the First Day of the Rest of Your Life." But affirmation-type reminders work for the less curmudgeonly.

Reminders can be visual, spoken, or otherwise. I don't remember to do things unless I can see them, so I keep multivitamins in a clear acrylic canister on the counter. A pretty bowl of fruit is a reminder of healthy snacks; conversely, less healthy snacks stay behind closed cabinets or in snack drawers or in a bank vault. Out of sight, out of mind.

Support

I have a relatively social job that puts me frequently at cocktail parties and schmoozefests. It takes a high level of energy and focus to be "on" all the time and affect a tinkly laugh. So when I'm off-duty, the last thing I want to do is attend a touchy-feely group meeting. But I was astonished at how effective it was when my readers responded each week with e-mails. A few became pals. Irwin hectored me: "Give up sugar! You're kidding yourself!" Linda and Ethel were funny and supportive. James was patient; all his e-mails arrived with the slug line "Continue to go for it." I liked seeing that phrase in my in-box; dare I call it an affirmation? Grounding yourself in other people's stories and getting a guaranteed stream of encouragement is a psychological tonic that goes beyond the immediacy of the structure it provides.

Support groups help in ways that can't be quantified. They're crucial to the success of Weight Watchers. They're essential to Linda, who went from dreading the "strangers" at her AA group to referring to the rest of the world as "civilians," outsiders. The breast-cancer support group I attended during my treatments in 1996 was the only place where I felt comfortable expressing my resentment of people with a full head of hair.

★ Value-Added Tax

A friend of Ethel's always kids that he'll find her a guy if she pays him $10,000 to do it. When he saw how much weight she'd lost, she told me, "he said he's lowering his price to $7,500 because I'm thinner now and more marketable."

If group meetings aren't convenient or just not your thing, or if you're terribly famous and don't want to spend your time signing autographs, you can get the same support effect online or by telephone.

One day when I was feeling sorry for myself about this endless weight-loss thing, the newspaper vendor on my corner recognized me as I trudged dejectedly to the gym. "You're the one losing weight!" he called out. "Keep it up, you're doing it for all of us!" He grabbed a piece of his gut and wiggled it in solidarity. Thereafter, whenever I saw him on the corner, I'd speed up and pretend to run, triumphant, as if finishing a marathon; we both enjoyed the joke and it was a daily ritual to look forward to.

Alas, my gut-waggling vendor was transferred to another corner, and the replacement vendor seems to have as many screws loose as teeth. It's like in *Annie Hall* where Woody Allen tries to share the same joke about lobsters amok in the kitchen with a new girlfriend, but she's no Diane Keaton. The joke dies with the end of the relationship.

Still, the corner itself has come to represent my anonymous friend, the vendor with the high-fives and the pinch-an-inch greeting. I always feel heartened when I pass that corner; good vibes rubbed off on me there like fresh newsprint.

Support can come from such unlikely places as your street corner. It can come from the homeless man I passed the other day—I know, not all communities offer weight-loss support from the homeless sector—who commented, after I passed without giving him any spare change, "Anyway, you have nice legs."

There was a time when I bridled at compliments like that, but I was secretly thrilled. I mean, I *do* have nice legs!

★ Compliments, a Minefield

Some people think it's polite or even clever to compliment fat people on losing weight even when it's clear they haven't. Perhaps it's meant as a subliminal prod in the right direction.

But the fat aren't fooled by this enormously condescending ruse. I had a neighbor who must have read somewhere that this is what women want. He'd squint at me as if he'd discovered a new planet in the solar system and ask in hushed tones—as if it's an awesome secret just between the two of us—*"Is it my imagination or have you lost weight?"*

It's your imagination, you moron, and you asked me the same thing only yesterday.

When you're losing weight, you're touchy about who says what. Of course you want people to notice, but compliments can be loaded, if not slightly insulting. If I look "terrific" now, what did you think of me before?

Then there's the pressure. If I lose 10 pounds and everyone loves me for it, what if I gain it back (as about 97 percent of dieters do) and the praise dries up? Where are those compliments now? All you see are tight, prim lips and embarrassment where before there were promises of a confetti parade up the Canyon of Heroes.

I have plenty of supportive friends, and my sister calls in almost daily for progress updates. (When I go off the rails she makes a sound deep in her throat like the warning growl of territorial cats.) Nevertheless, the relatively anonymity of group support can help in ways you can't replicate with people who know you too well to be dispassionate and objective. Friends might cut you slack when they shouldn't or be too hard on you when they should back off. They press your buttons. Simmering grievances and jealousies can get in the way; a small slice of my weight-gain pie went to trying to keep the peace with girlfriends who felt competitive with me over men or career. It makes me angry now to realize how I unconsciously tried to appear less threatening to them by abusing my body; in the future, I'd sooner give up a friendship like that than my power. (Anyway, it's counter-intuitive to make yourself seem smaller by making yourself fatter.)

When I was sixteen, like most girls that age, I began obsessing in earnest about my size, even though I was a normal weight. All that body anxiety was coming from elsewhere—budding sexuality, peer pressure, social insecurity. After hearing my endless litany of woes—"I'm fat! I'm too fat!"—my mother snapped at me. "You're getting boring," she said.

Doubtless it was true. It's fabulously boring to hear others complain about being overweight when they're not. It was like a slap in the face all the same; if your own *mother* thinks you're boring, is there any hope?

I can see now that I was nervous about the attention my body was getting. The fear of having a womanly body and all the expectations and responsibilities that come with it can trigger anorexia at that age. When I wailed about gaining weight, I wasn't fishing for compliments or sympathy; I was looking for reassurance that I'd be safe and protected. My burgeoning curves were on display in school, on the street, in the park, and I experienced it as harmful, a terrifying loss of control after a childhood in which a few dicey incidents had already muddied the waters.

How was my mother to know this? Even *I* didn't know this. Family and friends see you a certain way, their perception bolstered by the facts of their history with you. You can grow up to be a crack ho and they'll still remember you playing with your dollies.

Support implies encouragement. Again, family and friends can prove deadly here. A good friend is an honest friend, but sometimes brutal honesty can kill your dreams. At the same time, you don't want to depend on fawning friends who tell you how *super* you are. If they whitewash the truth, how can you trust anything they say?

The best support is the buddy system—preferably more than one buddy—one or more friends or acquaintances you can turn to as different needs arise. You might need a pep talk one day and a smackdown the next.

The buddy system is invaluable when it's a buddy who's in the same boat. Amanda the Exercise Nazi doesn't have a weight problem, but she's dedicated to a life of physical health. Any visit with her will necessarily involve aerobics *à deux*. You need to be able to turn to someone who'll do what you're doing, side by side. Dine with friends who likewise order their fish broiled with lemon. Make a date with a skiing buddy to ski, with a walking buddy to walk. Without Diane Stefani meeting me three to five mornings each week, my gym ID card would have been the plastic I use to jimmy open doors when I've locked myself out.

I'm a buddy slut. When I *really* need volunteers to babysit me at the gym, I throw myself at their feet. I ran into Maralyn at JoAnne's birthday party years after we'd last been in contact. Maralyn had moved out of the city to a place right near a horse stable and mentioned she was taking lessons.

"I *love* riding!" I said.

"Well, you certainly must come out sometime," said Maralyn. Maybe she meant it politely, a conversational tic. But you know what? I didn't care! The next day I was on the phone scheduling horseback-riding dates for the summer. Maralyn already had a regular riding buddy, but I wasn't too proud to tag along.

Structure

People think because I work from home and have written a string of books while holding a day job that I must be incredibly disciplined by nature. *Not!* I can assure you I didn't come by self-discipline naturally; it's still a work in progress.

Even when I'm able to hunker down and get enormous quantities of work done—ten hours at a stretch with a laptop propped on my knees until I've ossified—I spin my wheels more than necessary. The problem: No structure. Going for the world record in typing from an awkward position on the couch isn't ultimately as useful as scheduling work in sensible two-hour bites broken up by exercise, phone calls, or practicing piano.

Cross-training for business, I call it. But I rarely do it.

Discipline, like weight loss, isn't about willpower. It's not about stamina and feats of endurance. Discipline is about behavior that unfolds within a framework. When the framework is solid and adapted to your lifestyle (Do you have to get the kids to school? Are you a gunrunner with a crazy schedule, always living out of suitcases or in a prison cell?), *then* work gets done.

Healthy living requires a framework as well, a sense of when to eat, how much to eat, where to fit in exercise, how to measure progress. For my weight loss I built a framework piece by piece. You'll probably want me over for your next barn raising.

For most people, or for beginners at weight loss, a ready-made structure is often a more viable solution—at least at first. You want someone else to develop the lesson plan and hand out the coursework, someone to bark at you that at precisely 10:37 A.M. you're to unwrap your cheese-and-apple snack as if you were on the *Mission: Impossible* team and it was time to lay out the tools to wiretap the drug lord's phone. The wide world of food choices is a quandary for someone who isn't sure which tie goes with which shirt.

There's nothing wrong with signing up for a commercial weight-loss plan that provides a basic structure you can use as a template while you consider what parts of it work best for you. If you recall the government website I mentioned earlier that counts how many calories you expend by removing slag, you'll realize that the slag removers probably have different lifestyle requirements from those of the animal butchers.

A workable structure is a blueprint for how to lose weight on a day-to-day basis. It doesn't need to be anything so formal as a written schedule (although that's nice when you're starting out), because after a while it should be automatic, just the way you once reached mindlessly for Twinkies.

★ Throw It Away

The more times you resist a particular food craving, the easier it gets. But that first time is a bitch.

To start, try throwing something away. Not your firstborn, but something nearly as beloved—a chocolate bar or a bag of chips, say. Whatever floats your boat, or just bloats you.

In a ceremony that might've gotten us burned as witches in Salem, my friends and I threw away tokens of our favorite foods. Regretfully, I consigned a York Peppermint Pattie to the trash. Breaking up is hard to do! Then we sat in a circle and discussed it as if we were at a bereavement support group.

Studies show that 97 percent of women have cravings, mostly for fat, sugar, and endorphin-yielding foods like chocolate. Men are 68 percent subject to cravings and tend to prefer chips, preferably with a TV remote in the other hand.

Can behavior like this ever become a second skin, even if you were raised on Coca-Cola in your baby bottle? As recently as after losing

60 pounds, I would have said no, that you can't go back and make up for what you didn't get in childhood. I would have argued that you can train yourself anew but it'll never come naturally, you'd always have to remind yourself and live with the specter of relapse.

But now I'm thinking . . . *yes.* You can truly replace bad habits with good ones. I can see it in how I became an early riser, how I can go months without eating or craving my prime trigger foods, how even when I overeat I'm painfully aware of it.

Why did I succeed with those behaviors and not with others, equally important? Why isn't meal planning second nature to me?

Because I worked harder and more consistently on some areas until they took on a life of their own while leaving other behaviors on the back burner. My journey isn't over.

There's organizing the structure, and then there's living it. The organizing part is fun. I like to apply a tip I got from *Organizing from the Inside Out,* by Julie Morgenstern, about how to create an environment that hums along efficiently. Look around and ask yourself: What works? What doesn't?

Mealtimes should be as regular and predictable as you can make them. But I can't count on breakfast before my workout, because sometimes I'm out the door way too early for a bowl of cornflakes. Breakfast as the first order of the day sounds like a good idea, but . . . *it doesn't work for me,* at least not every day. My structure regarding breakfast has to be flexible, and often I divide up breakfast into little pieces—an apple before my workout and a bowl of oatmeal afterward, for example.

Healthy snacks between meals are important for taking the edge off hunger. They also break up the day, acting like a light at the end of the tunnel. But I'm not allowed to bring food into screening rooms; I can't yell to the projectionist, "Stop the film! We already know the chick is a guy! I'm having a yogurt!" My daytime snacks need to be planned in advance, but they happen at different times of the day, depending on my schedule.

Precision planning is helpful, but for me . . . *it doesn't work.*

Structure isn't synonymous with prison. Make it flexible and creative. Tailor it to contingencies.

Structure is also about behavior. Here's a supporting pillar of my structure: When I go to a Japanese restaurant, I order sushi or sashimi. It's a law, like waiting for the green light before crossing the street. I don't look at menus in Japanese restaurants because I don't want my head turned by the words *teriyaki* (sweet and sticky) or *tempura* (battered and fried); it's sushi or sashimi, and that's that.

A behavioral law of this sort is something I developed after I saw what didn't work. When friends met me for dinner on the spur of the moment, I often couldn't process the menu selections quickly enough to make healthy choices. You don't want to leave your friends hanging while you study the appetizers as if they were the Dead Sea Scrolls. I needed a few restaurants or dishes that were "safe," no-brainers. Now when a dinner companion suggests I choose the place, I don't let my mind roam to Artisanal, a restaurant that specializes in cheese—like going to Grindelwald without the commute—or the House of Well-Marbled Steaks. "How about Japanese?" I'll say. When I get there, the menu lies unopened.

The sushi-sashimi rule is part of my overall structure, something that never fails to work. I trot it out when necessary, when the strain of decision making in restaurants is more than I can handle.

★ Learn the Lingo

Reading food labels and claims is like deciphering the Rosetta Stone, but it's worth learning this tricky language because so many buzzwords are deliberately misleading. Take, for instance, the pursuit of a healthy loaf of bread. Here's one that seems to promise the benefits of grain, yet the word *grain* in itself doesn't mean "healthy." *Multigrain* (or *seven-grain*) doesn't necessarily mean "whole," *whole-grain* doesn't necessarily mean "100 percent whole-grain," and *made with whole grain* could mean there's one whole grain sitting like a cherry on top of a heap of refined flour.

Planning

Figuring out meals and shopping lists ahead of time is only part of the planning process. You also need to reassess your progress and goals at frequent intervals, since they change along with your clothing size. An initial goal might have been: I want to come out of hiding. That goal is beside the point once you're dancing on tabletops at the kind of bar where bras hang from the rafters.

Strategies change with the seasons or special occasions. Getting ready for bathing-suit weather is different from trying to make it through the gauntlet of holiday parties in one piece. Summer might be mostly about the calories, whereas winter might depend on behavioral flourishes—like arriving late to parties or leaving early to minimize exposure to finger food.

Along with your finances, weight-loss goals should have short-, medium-, and long-range strategies, a pie chart of behaviors that curtail risk.

Let's say you plan to go to the gym tomorrow. Good idea. But have you mapped out how to accomplish it? Making a date with a gym buddy and setting the alarm early weren't enough for me. Getting out the door at an hour when my brain was still officially Closed for Business was slow going, so the night before, I'd lay out my gym clothes, iPod, keys, water bottle, gym lock, and membership card. I would heap it all on the floor by the bed. And I would set the timer on the coffeemaker Marie's mom had sent me so that by the time the alarm went off, the percolating was well under way. I'd become a Looney Toons character, my body floating through the air on coffee fumes toward the source.

★ Restaurant Desserts

Problem: When I go out to dinner with friends everyone orders dessert. And don't tell me to order fruit.

Solution: *Order fruit*. Come on, don't be a baby. Or else nurse a skim cappuccino whose foamy top is a distant cousin to whipped cream. Or pretend to receive a text message from Brad Pitt: He needs to see you right away. Politely excuse yourself; your friends will understand.

Planning is multipronged. You should have as many plans for different situations as you used to have excuses for why you couldn't possibly change your ways.

Consider dining out. You should have at your fingertips a list of "safe" restaurants where you don't have to study the menu like a map of Aztec treasure to figure out what isn't fried. You should go into restaurants armed with a policy of not ordering resolve-killing alcohol until after you've ordered food. Your dining-out strategies could include always taking home half of whatever you order, having a second appetizer instead of a main course, always starting with salad or a noncreamy soup, and, if you *must* have dessert, sharing it.

Is it too much to ask that you treat the breadbasket as a nonedible table ornament? Yes, I suppose it is.

It's a good idea to develop a package of plans for all the difficult scenarios you expect in the coming week: Stressful days. Meals on the run.

Vacation. Working late. Planning doesn't ensure perfection, but the goal is to increase your chances of doing better than before. That won't happen if you fly by the seat of your elastic-waist pants.

Measure

How do you *know* if you've done better than before? By measuring your progress. The number on the scale is one measure, and even though it's overused, numbers like that are psychologically appealing. They're clean, simple, iconic. Other numbered measures include body dimensions, clothing sizes, how many repetitions you can do with a dumbbell, the poundage you can lift, the distance you can run, the time it takes to do it.

Numbers have a place in your quiver. So do other forms of measurement: how clothes *fit,* how you *feel.* Small improvements in stamina.

Journal, like *juice,* isn't a verb . . . but we won't get into that again, it will only make my blood pressure jump. Looking back through your notes can remind you of the leaps and bounds you've made. I was startled to read in my journal about taking a cab to pick up a car that was at a garage only half a mile away; today I'd never waste money on a cab in good weather just to avoid a 5-minute walk.

Bite-sized Philosophies

Also known as attitude adjustment, this is where you craft the philosophies you wish to live by. Though not a fan of gooey affirmations, I well understand the power of words. So if you've been greeting the day with "I'm a fat, lazy slug!," now's a good time to switch to "I'm a person who lives life to the fullest," or something less boastful.

If you've seen me muttering under my breath on the street, you might catch this fragment: "I'm a person who loves to take public transportation." At first, that was wishful thinking. I didn't prefer public transportation—

I preferred *taxis*—until I bought an unlimited subway card and began to experience the thrill of the (nearly) free ride. The more I use the card, the less each ride costs.

Granted, this is a small thrill. But I can't help it; I love the idea that I'm sticking it to The Man! And I love running up and down subway stairs several times a day as a built-in form of exercise that has become an unremarkable part of my life. I may have started out muttering under false pretenses about public transportation, but it became true. I may have to change it in the future to: I love *walking* everywhere instead of taking public transportation. Maybe it will happen.

A mini-philosophy doesn't have to be true at the outset, just something you're striving for. We all have ideas about who we are, but many of these ideas are overly harsh and pessimistic, embedded in the subconscious at an early age and gnarling up the root structure of the brain. Unlike goals, which can be helpful even when phrased as a negative, your philosophy of yourself should be positive without being ludicrous. "I am queen of all I survey" is a bit much. "I'm a person who likes to learn from my mistakes" might sound like a Cinderella dream, but Cinderella managed to get to the ball and have a good time despite the curfew.

Accountability

You can run, but you can't hide. Or maybe you *can't* run because it makes you wheeze, but in any case you *still* can't hide.

Deceit won't help you lose weight. When I fell off that bike on the Hudson River path, my slow recovery time, shortness of breath, feelings of panic and nausea, and damp palms announced to the world that I wasn't in shape. No matter that I was doing something active, wearing athletic-looking clothing, and working up a sweat. I was the only person surprised at my lack of fitness because I still entertained the idea that the fitness I enjoyed as a child, teen, and young adult was mine forever. But at

230 pounds you can't just hop on a bike one afternoon and make up for years of neglect.

Accountability means checking in with friends, charting your weight loss, keeping a food diary, and keeping a journal that underscores connections between food and behavior with startling clarity. Let's see, I lost my job and ate a pie. I got bad news at the doctor and bought the Halloween-size bag of Snickers. Is there . . . could there be . . . a *connection?*

Shining the light of truth on what you're doing keeps you honest. I sometimes wished my friends would get together and perform a calorie intervention similar to what is done for alcoholics. "Tough love time," I'd imagine them saying. "Go get help or we won't meet you for brunch." JoAnne actually called my primary care physician to confide her fears about how breathless I was getting during our weekly walks over the Brooklyn Bridge.

But it's your move, not theirs. Should your friends wire your jaw shut? Are they licensed to do that? Have they sterilized the equipment?

When I'm in trouble I call the Nutrition Twins, and the first thing they do is demand to see a daily food diary. This simple act of accountability makes it less likely I'll eat something too embarrassing to document.

Keeping a food diary is a must. Unfortunately, I hate it.

Oh, how I hate it. I write for a living, but this is one thing I don't like to write. I pretend I don't need it, it's too bothersome, it's not all it's cracked up to be—rationalizations that are part of the same old subterfuge. My intense aversion to writing everything down and owning up to what I eat is proof of how powerful it is to come clean.

Motivational Shortcuts

Most people are familiar with basic tricks of the trade, like eating dinner off a salad plate to give the illusion of groaning abundance or eating with chopsticks to slow you down.

According to Amy O'Connor, deputy editor at *Prevention* magazine, your plates should be blue, your kitchen bright, and your workout area full of peppermint-scented candles. Athletes who inhaled peppermint did more sit-ups. People who ate off small blue plates (the Blue Plate Special?) ate considerably less than those dipping into the trough.

Reward yourself, but not with food. Take a bubble bath, see a movie, get yourself a boy toy. If you're wealthy, buy yourself a villa in the South of France every time you politely refuse seconds.

The annoying self-esteem movement flings kudos like grains of rice at a wedding—*You only murdered five people this week. That's such an improvement!* Rewards for weight loss should be based on legitimate accomplishments or they become meaningless.

Rewards are one kind of motivation. Fill your life with others: reminders (a nutrition book is on my bedside table), behaviors (I've moved the "safe" takeout menus to the top of the pile), tantalizing promises (taking a clothing inventory gives you an idea of what you can buy next).

JoAnne likes to run. She motivates herself to run faster and longer by cramming her iPod with songs that speak to her even when they're—by her own account—corny. She's got "Know Where I've Been," from the musical *Hairspray,* because "civil rights does it for me, baby!"

JoAnne's Playlist

When JoAnne goes running she needs inspiration on her iPod from the corny to the rockin'. Here's her somewhat apologetic, personally annotated playlist:

"Chariots of Fire" theme song
(I'm running! I'm running!)

"My Sharona"

"Golddigger"

"Pass That Dutch"

"I Will Survive"

"Thunder Road"

"Smiling Faces Sometimes"

"These Boots Were Made for Walkin'" (Jessica Simpson version; I'm not kidding!)

"Candy Shop" (50 Cent . . . Sexy . . .)

"All in Love Is Fair"

"Back on the Chain Gang"

"Your Mama Don't Dance"

"It's Raining Men"

"Roxanne"

"Pump It"

"Mandy" (For that, I'm really sorry.)

"Do Somethin'" (It's Britney, I know. Again, I'm sorry.)

"The Impossible Dream" (*Sob!*)

"I Know Where I've Been"

"Brown Sugar"

"Walking in Memphis" (My current fave.)

"I Am What I Am"

"Brand New Day" (Helps me stay married.)

"Desert Rose"

"Eye of the Tiger" (Bring it on, Rocky!)

"I Finally Found Someone"

"The Bitch Is Back"

"Stacy's Mom"

"Young Girl" (Reminds me of when I was fourteen.)

"Up on the Roof"

"It's All Coming Back to Me"

"Holla Back Girl"

"Every Little Thing She Does Is Magic"

"Shark Tale" theme song (cool girls singing)

"Let's Dance" (Makes me happy.)

"Lady"

"Where Is the Love?"

"Enough Is Enough (No More Tears)"

"Seasons of Love"

"Play That Funky Music"

"Rocky Mountain High" (I'm *sooo* embarrassed.)

"Annie's Song" (ditto)

Fine-tuning

I usually call this micromanaging, and not in an altogether complimentary way. It's true that grapefruit can be good for the digestion (although not when taken with certain meds), and that pairing rice with beans is a happy nutritional marriage.

Knowing such tricks is laudable. But organizing your life around infinitesimal improvements can become obsessive if not pointless. I know this from experience: After I first started weight training at 190 pounds when I was on my way up the scale, I called my trainer, Norman, from vacation with an emergency question: Should I put butter or jam on my toast?

I don't remember what he answered. He was probably mystified by the phone call. In any case, as someone who'd never been fat in his life, Norman's idea of breakfast is bacon; *"burn the shit out of it"* is how he orders it in restaurants. Such a nice Bronx boy.

I was trying to learn to choose my foods carefully, but the butter-jam question, at least under these circumstances, was impossible to answer and not worth the effort. Pats of restaurant butter are 40 calories, and in my extensive experience one of those butter pats covers pretty much nothing, hardly a corner of toast. You probably think you're being "good" by choosing those watery jam lozenges, so you help yourself to a few packets, but they don't carry nutritional content on their miniature packaging, and unless they're sugar-free, they pack just as many calories as the butter pat. By helping yourself to several of them, you wind up consuming more calories than if you'd stuck with the butter you wanted in the first place.

So don't get insane. Don't pull out spreadsheets in the middle of the restaurant. Don't call your trainer on Sunday morning at 8 A.M. for a whispered discussion of your hotel's breakfast buffet. Do what my friend Ethel does when she jots down how much peanut butter she had that day: "A *schmear* is a measurement, right?"

★ Milking It

The dairy industry, like the meat industry, has powerful lobbyists. If you were working for the USDA, would you rather be schmoozed by the dairy folk at an all-night fondue fest or sit on a park bench for a supper of sprouts with Concerned People for Digging Your Food from the Ground by the Roots?

All that hobnobbing might explain why the Food Pyramid traditionally presents meat and dairy as integral to a balanced diet (when Asians on cheese-less fish diets are the ones who tend to live longer).

Recently, the milk men claimed that dairy products help you lose weight. This assertion is based on three studies by a researcher with a patent on his claim (and whose work was financed by the Dairy Council), and it says that eating dairy products three times a day can make you slim. The researcher looked at a total of only 46 people, and the first study lacked a control group. The fine print also raises suspicions: It worked only for people who were already overweight, ate too much, and had low calcium and protein intake.

Two subsequent studies by independent researchers rejected those findings. As this book goes to press, the Federal Trade Commission is reviewing ads making that weight-loss claim and the Physicians Committee for Responsible Medicine is suing three dairy trade associations and a handful of companies for deceptive advertising.

I love cheese. I'm not giving it up. Neither do I kid myself that the high fat in a lovely St. André—or even the lower fat in some yogurts—will help me lose weight unless I eat it responsibly.

Yes, Ethel, a schmear is preferable to a perfectionist's panic attack.

Doing what you can to lose weight is good. Splitting hairs is a drag—*how many grains over half a cup of brown rice was that?* It's this kind of micromanaging that accounts for people following the letter, not the spirit, of the Glycemic Index, for example, and why people say, Hey, the Mediterranean Diet is healthy—I'll interpret that to mean I can drink all the wine I want with dinner!

There's only a small degree of play when controlling your weight on a daily basis. You can't alter your genetics or grow taller. You can't go back in time and start over. Meanwhile, by monkeying with caloric minutiae, you might be missing out on the calorie-burning bonanza of increased muscle mass. Micromanagers see exercise in terms of burning off exactly enough calories to cheat with at dessert. Fine-tuners see it as building a nest egg.

Don't Make Fun of My Diet Pepsi

There's always some joker who snickers when I order a diet drink with my food. They think I'm deluding myself that the soda will magically suck the calories out of my meal and render them harmless.

Har har, I get it.

But I'm right to order diet drinks. A 12-ounce can of regular Coke has *9 teaspoons of sugar*. So if I want a cheeseburger—and sometimes I do— are you telling me that for the sake of propriety I should also consume a heaping glass of sugar-water? One sugared soda a day gives you an extra 1000 calories a week. In a year, that's . . . *15 pounds*.

If you do nothing different in your daily life, you'll gain weight. It's the inevitable result of the aging process, which robs you of muscle mass over the years. With less muscle, you burn fewer calories. Fortunately, studies prove you can increase muscle at any age, even if you're in a wheelchair in a nursing home (believe it or not, that's when you can most benefit). A lot of people in nursing homes are only there because they don't have the strength to get out of a chair, not because of any mental impairment or debilitating disease.

There are only so many calories a person can cut from the diet. But if you raise your metabolism through adding muscle, the body burns more calories 24/7. Why agonize over butter versus jam when you can be turning your body into a fat-burning machine?

Make Mine Mini

Buy individual portions of food. Make a special trip when you want a low-fat frozen dessert, get the smallest size, and eat it there. JoAnne will walk miles for Tasti D-Lite, which, rap-style, she calls Tasti D's. Philadelphia Cream Cheese is sold in packs of individual servings, just enough to spread on two pieces of whole-wheat toast.

My previous idea of a portion is whatever happened to be on my plate. If it's a spoonful, I eat it, and it's enough. If it's like the mountain of mashed potatoes Richard Dreyfuss toyed with in *Close Encounters of the Third Kind,* so be it.

I now know what portions are *supposed* to look like—the 9-volt battery of cheese, the deck of cards of chicken breast. But I have trouble leaving food on my plate, so I buy individual portions when possible. They tend to cost more, but not in the long run, once you account for how much you overspend when you overeat.

Keep It in Perspective

Bob Wright likes to tell a joke about the guy who passes a construction site where a religious building is going up. There are three hardhats working there. He says to the first one, "What are you doing?" The workman replies, "I'm mixing cement." The man moves farther along the site and comes across the second hardhat. Again he asks, "What are you doing?" The guy says, "Well, I'm just laying some bricks." Farther down there's another worker and it looks like he's got the worst job of all,

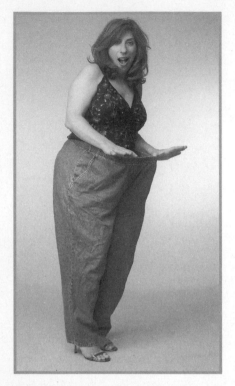

Where'd it all go? If Scarlett O'Hara could make a dress from her drapes, I could probably make drapes from my size 26 Fat Pants, which have so much elastic they could have kept the New Orleans levees together. (*Photo by Steve Brickles.*)

hauling bricks across the site. The man asks, "And what are *you* doing?"

The hardhat replies, "Me? I'm building a cathedral."

★

After three years of steady but modest weight loss, I got to a size 12—although when this photo was taken I was still flirting with 14s. Here I'm wearing a red-sequined Sean John top and my first ever pair of Jimmy Choo sandals. While they don't show to best advantage when paired with the Fat Pants, I hopped around ecstatically during the photo shoot and was happy to pose for photographer Steve Brickles with a look of pleased shock, as if 75 pounds had crept away of their own accord. See, weight loss can be fun!

For someone like me, maintaining a healthy weight will be a lifelong project. I'm not unhappy about that now that I have the knowledge and skills to keep it going. And there are the usual perks along the way: nicer clothes, increased body awareness, and a pair of Jimmy Choo high heels that are a far cry from the "comfortable shoes" I wore to an office party once, where my friend Denise took me aside and said, "Don't ever let me catch you wearing those ugly-ass shoes again!"

But at the end of the day, taking care of yourself, like kindness to strangers and generosity of spirit, is its own reward.

THE Cook   Fall 1969   8th grade 13 yrs old

Once, I had a problem weighty, when the scale hit hundred eighty
Caused by many a meal, and curious sauces with rich food galore
While I readied for meat tearing, suddenly, the Cook was swearing.
But, (as I was hard of hearing) I did not know Cook had swore.
"Meat's delicious", I muttered, nibbling at an apple core.
        The Cook said, "Please, eat nothing more".

Ah, distinctly, I recall, it was in the early fall,
And each separate dining hall left its bill upon my floor.
Eagerly the Cook was hired; so much eating left me tired.
Soon my scale and I grew spastic searching for a good domestic.
So, I settled for this maiden whom the butlers call "Igor".
        Need I tell you any more?

And the lumpy, bad, uncertain bowl of ~~tasted~~ tasteless sour brauten
Filled me - killed me with fantastic ulcers never felt before.
So that now - to still the dripping acid stomach, Cook stood repeating:
"Take the roast beef entreating entrance at your mouth and throw it on the floor.
        Watch your weight! Eat nothing more!"

As I watched, my stomach starving, Cook began the turkey carving.
Then the Cook began her raving, saying she could stand no more.
She watched me down the turkey carved, and then I ate potatoes. As I finished 12 tomatoes, Cook was
                        kicking on the floor.
"Get thee hence", I told the Cook. She left me, slamming my front door.
        Quoth my scale - three hundred four.

In the eighth grade, I wrote this parody of Edgar Allan Poe's "The Raven." No, it wasn't an act of prescience. The idea that fat would ever darken my doorstep was so absurd back then that the subject was fit only for satire.

CHEAT SHEET

Here's a summary of every pearl of wisdom in this book:

You can lose weight initially on any diet (but you'll have to segue into traditional low-fat, reduced-calorie eating to keep it off).

Lasting weight loss is about strategy, not willpower (plan for contingencies).

Stick to basics (don't play fast and loose with simple, tried-and-true rules).

Don't go to that party in the first place (if it's one of too many high-risk situations in your life).

Readiness comes by degrees (it's not all or nothing).

Embrace exercise at your pace and on your own terms (even if it means starting with a grumpy, resentful 5-minute walk).

Weight loss is a by-product of healthy living, not an end in itself.

People usually won't use a gym unless it's within four miles of home.

It's variety that makes an eating-and-exercise plan work.

Shock your body out of its rut by challenging it (if you want to see progress or break out of a plateau).

It's instructive to watch how thin people eat (look for reasonable role models).

Being connected to a healthy lifestyle to some degree at all times is more efficient in the long run than being "perfect" a fraction of the time.

Get rid of every single article of clothing that doesn't fit. (It's a leap of faith, but it frees you.)

Act as if you believe in yourself, and it will become so (nothing mystical here, just dime-store "as-if" psychology).

Accountability makes a difference (keep a daily food journal and show it to someone).

Cheese is a condiment. (I don't follow this as I should, but I see the point.)

Weight loss isn't about numbers, it's about change. (This is probably the hardest concept to grasp in a nation obsessed by scale panic.)

Maintenance includes setbacks. (There's no way around it, so learn from mistakes and move on.)

There's no substitute, or supplement, for the health benefits of a balanced diet. (Don't subscribe to wacko theories in the hopes of a shortcut.)

You've reached your goal not when the scale hits the sweet spot but when you embrace the behaviors it takes to keep it there.

Successful weight loss depends on eating a variety of foods in moderate portions, with an emphasis on low-fat and whole-grain, adding fitness, and losing weight slowly while making behavioral adjustments.

Learn to cook for yourself (there's no way to know what they're putting in your food at restaurants, but a good guess is oil, butter, and salt).

Take up activities you loved as a kid (you're more likely to stick with them).

Energy begets energy. (The more active you are, the more active you'll genuinely want to be.)

Sometimes to get to the tipping point you have to try everything at once. (Use as many strategies, tricks, and methods as you can instead of relying solely on calorie reduction or exercise.)

More: Accept a helping hand. Stop rationalizing. Be specific about your goals. Buddy up at the gym. Find creative ways to measure progress. Periodically reevaluate. Keep realistic expectations.

Unwise, better, best: Losing weight involves a series of choices along a sliding scale.

Degrees of "on": Ditto.

Practice.

GETTING STARTED
FLOW CHART

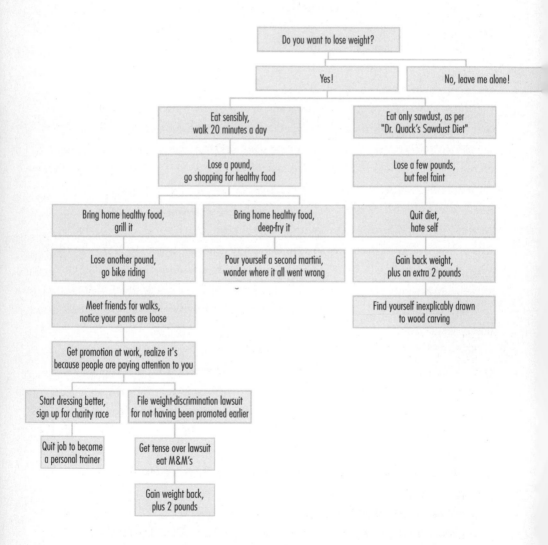

Do you want to lose weight?

Yes! → No, leave me alone!

Yes! branch:
Eat sensibly, walk 20 minutes a day

Lose a pound, go shopping for healthy food

- Bring home healthy food, grill it
- Bring home healthy food, deep-fry it

Bring home healthy food, grill it →
Lose another pound, go bike riding →
Meet friends for walks, notice your pants are loose →
Get promotion at work, realize it's because people are paying attention to you
- Start dressing better, sign up for charity race → Quit job to become a personal trainer
- File weight-discrimination lawsuit for not having been promoted earlier → Get tense over lawsuit, eat M&M's → Gain weight back, plus 2 pounds

Bring home healthy food, deep-fry it →
Pour yourself a second martini, wonder where it all went wrong

No, leave me alone! branch:
Eat only sawdust, as per "Dr. Quack's Sawdust Diet"

Lose a few pounds, but feel faint

Quit diet, hate self

Gain back weight, plus an extra 2 pounds

Find yourself inexplicably drawn to wood carving

ACKNOWLEDGMENTS

Just because I didn't follow a prescribed "diet" doesn't mean I did it all on my own. I had support and guidance from many sources, especially two couples: Diane Stefani and Terry Peikin, and Marie Menendez and George Sawicki. I shuttled between their households while I was waiting for installation at my new place of little amenities like "heat" and "walls." This manuscript was completed on their sofas and futons and AeroBeds. There were times when I polished off Terry's special ice cream or dipped into George's special pretzels—and don't ever mention the New Year's Eve truffle incident to Marie!—yet the friendships survived, my weight loss progressed, Diane and I got up every morning at 5:30 A.M. to make it to gym class, and my pets and I are eternally grateful for a place to warm our paws and keep our coats shiny.

My sister, Diane Bernard, vetted the chapter containing my childhood diary entries. "That was rough 'n' tough," she e-mailed after being reminded of some painful moments from our shared childhood, "but I understand why it's important that you include it, and I think you should." I love her for that, and for being my schwester.

My mom, Gloria, had naturally been afraid I'd spill all the family secrets. Mom, I only spilled a few. But while writing and thinking about the past, I gained an appreciation of how difficult her situation must have been, especially what with all the secrets I *didn't* spill.

A good friend is someone who gives it to you straight. When JoAnne Wasserman read an early chapter, she looked me in the eye and said, "This needs work." So I bitch-slapped her. *Kidding!* JoAnne helped me find my voice early on and we continue to take power-walks across the Brooklyn Bridge.

Good friends are hard to find and harder to keep. I keep mine chained in the basement so they won't get away: Marianne Goldstein, Stephanie Zacharek, Charles Taylor, Donna Dickman, Merrick Bursuk, Dorrie Crockett, Sue Pivnick, Maria Umali, Jack Mathews, and the Low family—Amanda, Peter, Charlie, Evan—were particularly helpful during my weight-loss process. I love all you guys to pieces.

My agent, Elaine Markson, thought I'd be a good fit with Megan Newman over at Penguin's Avery imprint. She was right. Megan was an absolute delight to work with—a sharp and funny editor, someone who "got" me immediately. Amazingly, she never doubted that I'd lose the weight as the book progressed; simply knowing I had her confidence made it that much easier.

At New York Health & Racquet Club, J. Travis made it his business to keep me motivated and on track. He got me hooked on Pablo Toribio's spin class and Anthony LaCagnina's magic massage. Lisa Schulman's bodysculpt classes gave me quads of steel and helped move me up to intermediate on the ski slopes.

J. also introduced me to the invaluable Nutrition Twins, Lyssie Lakatos and Tammy Lakotas Shames (www.nutritiontwins.com). They are angels who helped me out of many a tight spot (and waistband).

Iva Popovicova was my personal trainer through most of my weight loss, and later became a friend. We sometimes laugh so hard I think we shake off a pound on the spot.

Stephen Josephson gave me behavioral tips for dealing with setbacks. Chef Ian got me through my first Thanksgiving holiday without gaining weight. "Progress, not perfection," were among the words of wisdom from Lee Labrada, a fitness motivator and former Mr. Universe.

Hal and Kathie Aaron's annual ski trips were the least of what they did for me. They've changed my life by gradually expanding my universe of possibilities. They hooked me up with realtors extraordinaire Ann Bialek and Nick Guider of Halstead, and then with Stefani Bollag and Steve Miller at Merrill

Lynch, where my money now grows in inverse proportion to my body instead of the other way around.

No less important were fitness buddies and neighbors Helene Rutledge and Norman Bey, workouts and tips from fitness gurus Fred Hahn and Phil Campbell, and those sushi lunches with Gary Hill and Steve Beeman. Yoshi at John Masters Salon found me a hairstyle that, finally, I can be proud of.

I don't believe in quick weight loss, but let's face it—sometimes you have a dress you've gotta get into in a hurry. Evan Chacker helped me during a nail-biting deadline by using precepts from his "20-Day Challenge" program, in which you eat foods that make the body work harder to process. Evan's also a great personal trainer, and he helped me work out safely even after a whiplash accident.

I wouldn't have had a dress I had to get into in the first place without stylist Dorian May, who started me off on the happy, scary journey to my first new wardrobe at my shiny new weight. She's another one who gives it to you straight—her thoughtfully pursed lips told me that the gorgeous shoes I had my eye on weren't going to work, alas. "Ankle straps," she said, which is code in the world of nonmodels for "makes you look shorter."

And I wouldn't have needed a dress to get into in such a hurry if I hadn't been scheduled to shoot the cover photo for this book. Luckily, I found (through J. Travis, of course) the wonderful, patient, adorable Steve Brickles. He was more like a shrink than a photographer, fielding 3 A.M. panic calls: *Promise me you'll make me look good! Bring vodka!* On the day of the shoot, he put a cat in my lap to lower my blood pressure, and the rest of the session was a blast. With vodka. Also for that photo shoot, there was hairstylist Katy Does Hair, makeup by Margina Dennis, and eyebrows by Cristina Cruz of Kimara Ahnert.

After fending off wackos with their fad diets and high colonics, I found the voice of reason at Hilton Head Health Institute (www.hhhealth.com)—especially from Bob Wright and John Schmitz. They teach a medically and nutritionally sound program (sometimes tax deductible, too!) that closely echoes my core beliefs about safe-and-sane weight loss.

My faithful readers kept me motivated and on track far better than any tonic:

Ethel Wolvowitz, James Hulton, Irwin Leibowitz, Bill Garner, and Joe Crowell—and especially Linda Spear, who understood the deeper issues I was grappling with and gave generously of her time, personally and professionally.

Finally, and in some ways most important, since our days at Barnard College, Cyndi Stivers has been like the North Star of my professional life, guiding me past the undeniably rocky shoals of New York journalism.

INDEX

ABOUT THE AUTHOR

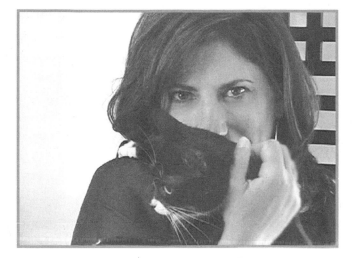

Jami Bernard is a film critic and author of books and social commentary. She is the first person to write a Lois Lane comic strip who ever worked in an actual newsroom, and her Lois is modeled on her own early days in journalism.

Jami shares her home with two cats and a twenty-one-year-old parrot who can whistle the theme from *Close Encounters of the Third Kind*.

For more information about Jami and updates on her weight loss, visit www.jamibernard.com.

362.196   Bernard, Jami.
B
          The incredible
            shrinking critic.

$22.95

DATE			

9/06